THE CUSP METHOD

THE CUSP METHOD

YOUR GUIDE TO BALANCED PORTIONS AND A HEALTHY LIFE

JACLYN DIGREGORIO

NEW DEGREE PRESS

THE CUSP METHOD

Your Guide to Balanced Portions and a Healthy Life

ISBN   978-1-5445-0010-2   *Paperback*

978-1-5445-0011-9   *Ebook*

CONTENTS

ABOUT THE AUTHOR

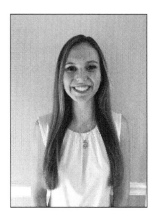 Jaclyn DiGregorio is the founder and CEO of CUSP Three Six Five, the first health and wellness brand to promote rule-free life-long nutrition.

As a certified fitness nutrition coach, Jaclyn developed the CUSP method while dealing with her own struggles with weight loss and dieting. As more and more people have begun to implement CUSP in their lives, CUSP Three Six Five was born to create tools that make her method simple to follow through the craziness of everyday life. Learn more at www.cuspthreesixfive.com.

Jaclyn loves all things nutrition, health and fitness. She is a proud finisher of the 2015 Marine Corps Marathon. Her favorite balanced meal consists of grilled salmon, mashed sweet potatoes, and oven roasted brussels sprouts. She is a 2017 graduate of Georgetown University's McDonough School of Business.

ACKNOWLEDGEMENTS

I am so incredibly thankful to everyone who helped make *The CUSP Method* possible. This magic could not have happened without Eric Koester, Shane Mac, Tucker Max, Jason Nellis, Dr. Susan Racette, Jeremy Brown and all my mentors. Thank you all for always pushing me to achieve the impossible. A million thanks to each of you for your extreme generosity and helping make my dreams become a reality.

To my editors, I cannot thank you enough for all of your time and wisdom. To my family—mom, dad, Rachel, Kevin, Christina and Keith—thank you for your endless love and support. Richie, thank you for always being my #1 fan. To my friends, thank you implementing CUSP into your own lives and showing the world how powerful this method can be. I love you all and do not know what I would do without you.

To the many amazing nutritionists, researchers, and college students who kindly gave me their time. This book would not have been possible without the powerful stories you graciously shared with me.

Most importantly, to the CUSP supporters, thank you for being passionate about a cause that is so important. Thank you for helping CUSP truly become a revolution in health.

INTRODUCTION

ONE GIRL'S STORY

I once knew a girl who exhibited many troubling behaviors. For the sake of anonymity, let's call her Jenny. Jenny was transitioning from high school to college. She was a petite and skinny girl who had a great metabolism. Jenny was athletic and played many sports. She came from a family that served healthy and balanced meals. It never really crossed her mind what she was going to eat because her mom always prepared her meals. Since she did not have to worry about her weight, she was never concerned with how much or how little she was eating. She simply listened to how hungry she felt and ate accordingly.

When she arrived at college, she was in an environment where so many of her friends, especially the females, were extremely concerned with their weight. She observed many girls who monitored everything they ate. Often these same girls were obsessed with exercising, and even though Jenny had never had a weight problem, she began to imitate their habits. She was at a time in her life when making friends was critical, and she wanted to fit in, not stand out. Trying to adjust to this new environment was enough of a challenge for Jenny. She had left her small town and knew no one on campus. It didn't even cross her mind that the habits she was forming were having negative effects on her body.

She didn't understand that by restricting herself from eating grains and only eating protein and vegetables, she was harming her metabolism. The extended periods of not eating always resulted in a high blood sugar spike as soon as Jenny ate anything. By exercising and then not eating a proper meal with the right types of macronutrients afterwards, she wasn't recovering from her workouts the way she was supposed to.

Sadly, it soon became a cycle in which Jenny would restrict her diet for as long as she could, and then she would crave all of the foods that she hadn't been allowing herself to eat. She would then overeat to the point that she felt sick. Jenny would have been lucky if the only adverse effects of these concerning behaviors were observed in her health, but unfortunately, they were more far-reaching. Her whole life began to spiral out of control. Jenny's grades dropped dramatically, she started losing friends, and she started disliking almost everything in her life and felt depressed. She could not attribute these changes to her extremely poor eating habits because she didn't realize that they had become so unhealthy.

Luckily, she started seeing a great nutritionist, and she learned about the positive effects of treating her body well. Jenny learned about what types of foods actually went into a balanced meal. She finally started allowing herself to eat all the treats that she had prohibited herself from having in the past, like pizza and cookies. By not restricting herself, she never overate, and she ended up losing the 27 pounds that she had gained. More importantly, Jenny never felt better! She was the happiest she had ever been. Jenny earned her best GPA of college, fell in love, ran a marathon, started her own business, and studied abroad in Italy (while eating pasta every day and still losing 8 pounds over one semester). So many positive things began coming her way, and it all was a result of a small change in her eating habits.

After watching Jenny struggle through tough times, I realized that she wasn't alone. I realized that this was a really serious problem on college campuses. I wanted to find out why these problems were occurring. I had a hunch that it had something to do with the environment of college campuses. If I was correct, I wanted to know how we can fix them, so I interviewed hundreds of college students, nutritionists and food researchers from across the country. Of the many students I interviewed, the ones referenced in this book have had their names changed to respect their privacy.

Oh and Jenny? That's me.

* * *

But here's the real truth — Jenny's happy ending (aka my happy ending), didn't come as easily as I made it seem. Yes, my story is true. I did meet weekly with an amazing registered dietitian, Allison Tepper. And yes, she gave me advice about many things, books to read and websites to visit. I credit her for most of my nutritional knowledge today. However, as great as it was to have someone helping me fill my toolbox with knowledge, there was no one who could apply these tools except me.

As I jumped back into my chaotic life and actually tried to use the skills I learned, I failed miserably. For nine long months, I constantly struggled. "If only I could find a simple way to win at the game," I used to think to myself. But I couldn't. It was too challenging and complicated. It seemed virtually impossible. I was on the verge of just giving up and accepting my unhealthy weight and dissatisfaction with life in general.

That was until one sunny, warm, mid-May morning when I found my secret weapon that I had been long searching for: portions.

It's not what you think, though. It was not meals in pre-sized containers and 100-calorie snacks. It was quite the opposite. It was, for the first time in my life, listening to my body. Instead of telling myself that I couldn't have the cookie or the french-fry, I told myself I could. Then, it was relying on my body's hunger cues to let me know when I had eaten enough cookies or french-fries.

This book reveals the secret that no one in the nutrition, diet and wellness space seems eager to talk about. It took everything I had inside of me to figure out a solution that would make it simple to eat healthy and be happy. And now, I want to share it with you, because your body deserves to be healthy, and you deserve to be happy.

In this book, you'll learn about my CUSP method, which is a super easy, foolproof method to simplify how I eat. It took me trial and error and months of failure after failure, but in the end for the first time since I can remember, I am not on a diet (yet I weigh less—funny how that works, right?) In fact, I eat whatever I want. I aim to incorporate balanced nutrition into every meal and most importantly, I portion my meals by listening to my body's internal cues.

What is CUSP? It's a simple acronym that you can take with you and apply no matter where you are.

Concentrate on what your body is in the mood for.

Understand which food types (fruits, veggies, protein or starch) make up the meal that you are in the mood for.

Supplement your meal with the food groups you are lacking.

Portion by listening to your body and following USDA's guidelines: ½ plate of fruits and veggies, ¼ plate of protein, and ¼ plate of starch.

CUSP aims to teach you how to approach real-life situations. My method will teach you how to make educated, healthy decisions, no matter where you are or who you are with. I know that we are humans and as much as we may aim for every single meal or snack that we consume to be balanced, there will be some days where we end up eating just a bowl of pasta for dinner, and that's okay. As long as we listen to our bodies to signal when we are satisfied (and thus, portion), the damage from that bowl of pasta will remain minimal.

Do you remember learning about cusps in high school math class? Depending on how long ago high school was for you or how present you actually were during class, you may need a refresher. Take a look at the graphic on the cover again. That's what a cusp looks like. Merriam-Webster defines cusp as, "a fixed point on a mathematical curve at which a point tracing the curve would exactly reverse its direction of motion." In other words, a cusp is the turning point. It's a point of transition.

The CUSP method is symbolic for my own turning point. Before I found my secret weapon, I was at an all-time low. By following the four steps of the CUSP method, I completely transformed my life. And it was so easy. I only wish that someone had told me this secret a few years sooner.

CUSP throws everything you've ever known about "dieting" in the trash. CUSP isn't just my turning point; it's a healthy turning point that I'm going to share with you.

And here's the best part, if it can survive the complexities of a college student's life, you can be sure it can handle pretty much anything you can throw at it. This book is beneficial for anyone. It can completely change your life and your relationship with your health, food and exercise. So pass it along to your mom, your grandma or your little brother after you finish.

Not only will this book help you become a healthier you, but it will also help contribute to a happier overall life. Other perks include: potential weight loss, increased confidence, meal ideas, skin improvement, higher quality sleep, increased productivity at work or at school, higher energy levels, and the ability to make a difference in the health of the people you love. I know that anyone who reads this book can transform his or her life the way I did.

I want you to feel those same levels of happiness that I currently hold in my heart, levels of happiness that I didn't even know were possible.

Welcome to the CUSP method...

PART 1

HOW WE GOT HERE

The research of Cornell University's Food and Brand Lab founder, Dr. Brian Wansink, is crucial to understanding why humans eat the way we do. Dr. Wansink has found the average person makes well over 200 food decisions on a daily basis. I can only consciously recall making about five yesterday (breakfast, lunch, dinner, and two snacks). So what causes us to make these decisions, especially if most of them are subconscious?

CHAPTER 1

THE "FINISH YOUR PLATE MENTALITY"

IN THIS CHAPTER YOU WILL LEARN:

- Why finishing your whole plate isn't always a good idea
- What you can do instead of finishing your whole plate
- Why it's so difficult to stop eating when food is in front of you
- The importance of portioning your plate so that you can finish all of the food in front of you and not worry about whether or not you overate
- How to handle portioning at a restaurant when you are served an XXL sized meal
- How to handle portioning at parties

* * *

"Taylor, you're not allowed to get up from the table until you finish your dinner!" Mrs. Wells shouted across the kitchen to her six-year-old daughter. "But Mom!!!!! All my friends are playing outside. I'm full." Taylor whined back to her mother. "Take three more bites of your chicken, and then you can join them." "Okay. Fine." Taylor moaned and forced three more bites of chicken down her throat, even though she already felt full.

Taylor recalled these memories to me as she was reflecting on the influences her childhood eating patterns have had on her current habits in college. She feels that there was definitely some sort of correlation with this forced finishing of her plate and her current lack of self-control when food is in front of her. The interaction Taylor described between her and her mother is unfortunately quite common.

During childhood even my parents, who are the most amazing parents in the whole world and will be reading this (hi mom and dad), would often require that I finished all of the food on my plate. It's easy to see why Mrs. Wells, my mom and many others, thought they were helping their children by encouraging this. Of course parents want to make sure their precious little boys and girls have enough to eat and most importantly, consume all of the nutrients their bodies need.

It's also common to feel guilty leaving food unfinished on a plate. I heard the comment, "There are starving children in Africa," made to someone who is throwing away perfectly good food more times than I can remember. I am saddened by the extreme poverty that sweeps the world we live in and the disturbing numbers of children who are starving. We can easily save the extra food on our plates as leftovers for a meal the next day. If we want to enact change and help the 795 million people who do not have enough food to live a healthy and active life, we can donate food, money or time to one of the many impressive nonprofits that strives to end this issue every single day. I'm not advocating that we ever waste food (as food waste is a huge problem on college campuses that we must tackle), but I am advocating for not finishing our plates if we already feel satisfied. Buy some Tupperware, and don't be afraid to take leftovers home at a restaurant.

In examining the issue from a parenting standpoint, I am excited and curious to see if this particular practice will start to change with millennials, like Taylor, becoming parents. If children are taught that they don't have to finish their plates, and they can stop eating when they are no longer hungry, maybe these habits will lessen how often they will overeat later in their lives. Although I'm hopeful that teaching children how to eat based on the way their bodies feel and not what's in front of them can go a long way, human nature kicks in at some point. It makes it difficult for us to stop eating if there is food in front of us, even if we are already full.

Internationally recognized nutritionist Dr. Lisa Young explained to me, "We're served portions that are big. Rather than eating with our stomach and stopping when we're full, we end up eating with our eyes based on what we see." It seems that if the food is in front of us, we often will eat it.

I asked Taylor to tell me more about this lack of self-control that she mentioned. She said there was no better way to illustrate it than to tell me the story of her dinner at an Italian restaurant last weekend. "Obviously I ordered pasta," she said. "I love fettuccine alfredo, and I had been looking forward to it all week. I knew the portion was enough to literally feed a family of four, and last time I went to this same restaurant, I finished the whole plate and felt pretty sick afterwards. I told myself I was only going to eat half and save the other half for lunch tomorrow. Then, I could enjoy it twice and not feel sick. But, I simply couldn't resist finishing the whole plate. I was with friends and the more we talked, the more distracted I became. I stopped thinking about what I was eating and before I knew it, I was ¾ of the way in. My stomach started to ache, and I again told myself I had eaten enough. As we sat and chatted for what seemed like hours, I ended up finishing all of the pasta."

It is clear that Taylor made an effort to become more aware of when she was full and should stop eating. Due to the way we are wired as human beings, it's extremely difficult to stop ourselves from eating food when it's sitting in front of us. It doesn't matter how hungry we are or what kind of food it is, we continue eating.

Dr. Wansink's bottomless soup bowl experiment illustrates that people eat what's in front of them and most of the time don't even realize how much they are actually eating. Students were invited to a special soup lunch where half of the attendees unknowingly ate out of self-refilling bowls. The results showed that those with the bottomless bowls ate 73% more soup. When asked how many calories they thought they consumed, the students estimated about the same as those eating out of the normal bowls.

Just like those students and Taylor, when food is in front of you, you'll probably eat it. It doesn't mean that you, Taylor or those students have weak willpower or can't control yourselves; it means you're just like everyone else. We are much better off attempting to reduce the amount of food we serve ourselves rather than trying to increase our self-control. This is why the P (portion) of the CUSP method is so important. If we portion our plates in a healthy way, it doesn't matter if we're preconditioned to finish them.

There are times, however, when a plate of food is in front of you, and there isn't much you can do about it. The odds are that most of the meals we order at restaurants will be XXL sized, just like Taylor's pasta plate. Even in situations like this, where you can't portion your own plate, you can still apply the CUSP method. Simply look at your plate before you begin to eat and decide how much of it you should portion for yourself.

Let's say you're at an Italian restaurant like Taylor and decide to order pizza because you are really craving it. (Concentrate on what your body is in the mood for.) Next, you think about what a regular pizza consists of, cheese and bread, which is protein and starch. (Understand what food types make up the meal that you are in the mood for.) You decide to add spinach and broccoli to your pizza. (Supplement your meal with the food groups you are lacking.)

Oh no, you hesitate. How can you possibly portion this pizza? It's going to be a huge portion served right in front of you, and just like Taylor, you're going to end up finishing your whole plate. Even if you try to portion it, the foods are all mixed together, how can you possibly figure out what ½ plate of veggies is? Don't worry! It doesn't have to be complicated at all. When your pizza arrives, roughly estimate the portion. There's no need to stress.

When you're out to eat and you're not portioning your own plate, it isn't going to be perfect. And that's okay, because by being aware of your portion and roughly how much is enough, you will avoid overeating and that's the key. And, just like anything else, practice makes perfect.

Estimating portions when you are out will become easier and easier the more you do it. For a personal pizza, I usually estimate a healthy portion size of about half of the plate. It's not the perfect ½ veggie, ¼ starch and ¼ protein combo that is ideal, but it does incorporate all three food groups and creates a portion that is not too large. Cut the pizza in half and plan to save the other half for the next day's lunch. (Portion by following USDA's guidelines.)

Also, remember to listen to your body. It will send you signals telling you that it is full and does not want any more food. The specific amount of food your body needs is different for everyone, but each of our bodies do tell us when we feel satisfied.

So what's next? You've eaten half of the pizza and you feel full and satisfied. But it's still sitting in front of you calling your name. Just like Taylor you are having trouble stopping yourself from overeating. Don't worry. I've been there. And luckily for you, I've figured out some tricks to stop you from overeating.

My favorite restaurant mind trick is to place my napkin on top of the food on my plate when I am already full and satisfied. Because I can no longer see the food sitting right in front of me, I'm much less likely to move the napkin and overeat. Out of sight, out of mind!

Another trick I have is chewing gum. Once the gum is in my mouth, I'm not too likely to want to eat more. I always keep a pack in my purse so that whenever I want to use this trick, I have a piece handy.

When I'm at a party, the struggle is usually the endless appetizers. No one likes ruining their appetite for dinner on appetizers, but we often fill up on cheese and crackers and regret it later. This is the same concept we've been discussing; the food is in front of you, so you eat it. If the party is at your place, try brushing your teeth with a minty toothpaste when you no longer want to eat. Works every time.

Luckily, at parties, you can fill up your own plate, unlike at most restaurants. If you only eat what's on your plate (portion), and you only serve yourself a balanced meal that you're in the mood for (concentrate, understand, supplement), you won't have to worry about being overfull from those appetizers by the time the meal is served. It all comes back to using the CUSP method every time you fill your plate.

* * *

CHANGES YOU CAN MAKE IN YOUR LIFE TODAY:

- If you are full and there is still food on your plate, don't eat it
  - Save it for a leftover

- ◆ Teach your children (or future children) to do the same
- When you have the opportunity to serve yourself, always portion your plate as close to the following guidelines as you can
  - ◆ ½ of your plate filled with veggies and or fruits
  - ◆ ¼ of your plate filled with starch
  - ◆ ¼ of your plate filled with protein
- When you're full at a restaurant and you are having trouble stopping yourself from overeating:
  - ◆ Place your napkin on top of your plate
  - ◆ Chew a piece of gum
- When you're at home and are having trouble stopping yourself from overeating
  - ◆ Brush your teeth with a minty toothpaste
- Pre-portion EVERYTHING—including snacks and desserts
  - ◆ One slice of cake will often turn into two slices unless you portion
  - ◆ Never, never eat from the bag or box of snacks, you'll quickly be wondering how the whole bag is already empty (I'm sure you already know this but just a friendly reminder)

CHAPTER 2

GROWING PORTIONS + GROWING PLATES = GROWING BELLIES

IN THIS CHAPTER YOU WILL LEARN:

- Just how much portions have grown since the 1950s (mentally prepare yourself for this one)
- Just how much plate size has grown since the 1950s (additional preparation needed here)
- How the size of our plates, bowls, and utensils influence how much we eat
- How to get the most (or more literally the least) out of our burger and fries (hint—portioning)

* * *

Every once in a while during Chelsea's childhood, her parents would take her out for a special treat. Mickey Dee's! What eight-year-old doesn't love a burger, fries, and a soda? What parent doesn't love a meal that you don't have to cook and that makes your child happy? (Come on—they call them happy meals for a reason.) Sure, fast food isn't the healthiest choice, but once in a while it can be a great treat. Everything in moderation, right?

We might find this to be true if we could jump in a time machine and go back to 1950. The Centers for Disease Control and Prevention (CDC) reported that an average fast food meal in the 1950s consisted of a 3.9-ounce hamburger, 2.4-ounce portion of french fries, and a 7-ounce soda. With those portion sizes, Chelsea's meal may have been lacking fruits and veggies, but in terms of calorie consumption, it wouldn't have been so bad.

Unfortunately, most fast food meals now have more calories than the average person needs in a day. The drastic increase in portion sizes disgusts me (about as much as the time when a cockroach crawled down my leg in the library, if not more). Dr. Young's research compares the portion sizes of fast food in 1950 to the portion sizes of those same foods today. She concluded that a 3.9-ounce hamburger from 1950 is now 12 ounces. Those 2.4-ounce fries are now 6.7 ounces. And the soda? A horrifying 500% growth brings that small 7-ounce treat to a whopping 42-ounces of sugary addiction.

The average adult today weighs 26 pounds more than the average adult weighed in 1950. I have a feeling those huge portions may have something to do with it.

Is it still okay to serve children fast food in moderation? This is something Chelsea will have to decide for herself as she told me she hopes to have children someday. If she wants to take her kids out for a fun and easy treat, fast food may no longer be just one unhealthy dinner. Instead, it's thousands of excess calories our bodies don't need. Who knows what fast food will be offering in the next 10 years. Considering the unprecedented growth during the past 66 years, it's a scary thought.

One option for Chelsea is to still allow her children to eat fast food (because it's important to teach them to concentrate on what their bodies are in the mood for), but to encourage that they split their fries or burger with her (because it's also important to teach them how to portion). This encourages eating the yummy fast food her children want, but not over-eating it.

Sadly, portion sizes aren't the only things that have grown dramatically since the 50s. Plate sizes have as well.

Chelsea's grandmother was eating off a 9-inch plate when she was a teenage girl, as that was the standard for the majority of ceramic dinner plates sold in the U.S at the time. Yet for some crazy reason, Chelsea's dinner plates are now 12 inches. Dr. Wansink and his colleague Dr. van Ittersum report a 36% increase in surface area of dinner plates since 1960.

Was Chelsea's grandmother less satisfied by her dinner because she was eating off a 9-inch plate? Absolutely not. Dr. Wansink, Dr. van Ittersum and their fellow researcher Dr. Painter studied the impact of changing the sizes of bowls and spoons to see how it would affect how much people ate and how much they thought they ate.

The researchers conducted their study at an ice cream social that was supposedly celebrating a colleague's achievement. All colleagues who attended the social were food and nutrition experts. Dr. Wansink, Dr. Ittersum and Dr. Painter were interested in seeing how these subtle changes in portions subconsciously affected even those most educated in the field. The results? People who were given larger bowls and spoons served themselves 53% more ice cream, and people who were given the larger bowls with regular spoons increased their serving size by 31%.

The worst part is, the participants didn't even realize they had served themselves more. It was actually the opposite effect.

The people with the smaller bowls were asked to estimate how much they had served themselves, and they ended up estimating that they had served themselves more than those with larger bowls (and a significantly larger amount of ice cream) due to the illusion of there being more ice cream in a smaller bowl.

Because it seems that there is more ice cream in a smaller bowl, the perception of satisfaction is much higher than a bigger bowl filled with the same amount of ice cream. This preconceived notion of future levels of satisfaction all occurs before the person even takes a single bite. The same applies to plates. Your meal appears bigger on a smaller plate, and you think you have eaten more than you actually have. Satisfaction is often based on how much you think you have eaten. It's the opposite with larger plates. Your meal appears smaller on a larger plate, and you begin to think, "Maybe this isn't enough for dinner" and instead eat more. The bigger plates, bowls, and utensils we use, the more food we serve ourselves.

Even if we aim to follow the C (concentrate), U (understand) and S (supplement) of CUSP, without the P (portion), we are stuck in that same cycle of overeating and restricting. And, with larger plates, bowls, and utensils, we make it hard on ourselves to follow the P and actually portion. Make it as easy as possible on yourself. Do not make it necessary to think twice about how much you're serving yourself. Upgrade your kitchen to smaller plates, bowls and utensils. You will be thankful for the simplicity it brings to portioning. And, if you are worried about the extra money this upgrade will cost, remember that every time you fill your plate with less food, that is less food you need to buy. What goes around will come back around many more times again.

* * *

CHANGES YOU CAN MAKE IN YOUR LIFE TODAY:

- Swap out the plates, bowls, and utensils in your kitchen for smaller ones
  - Aim for closer to 9 inches for your dinner plates (in comparison to the 12 or 13 inch ones you most likely have in your cabinet currently)
- If you are in the mood for fast food or takeout, remember you don't need to eat the whole burger, fries, and soda or shake meal by yourself
  - Try splitting the meal with a family member or friend
  - Substitute a side salad for fries

CHAPTER 3

THE IMPOSSIBLE CHALLENGE: ESTIMATING SERVING SIZE

___

IN THIS CHAPTER YOU WILL LEARN:

- Why humans have so much difficulty estimating serving size
- When recommended serving size is a good guideline and when to listen to your body instead
- The importance of keeping your kitchen stocked with serving measurement utensils at all times
- Why millennials may struggle more than other generations with estimating serving size
- How to estimate serving size with your hands for all those times when you're not in your own kitchen

* * *

Every once in a while (more often for some of us than others), we attempt to fill our plates or bowls with an appropriate serving of food. One student I interviewed, Mary, told me about her efforts to fill a bowl of ice cream with a portion large enough to satisfy her, but not too large that it would make her feel overfull. We've all felt both probably more than we would like to admit.

Mary decided to buy 1.5 quarts of Breyers Oreo Cookies & Cream flavored ice cream. She knew that she would have to create her own serving. Mary looked at the serving on the back of the package. "Only 130 calories for ice cream! Wow, that's not so bad," she thought to herself. The first problem to address here is that serving labels don't always mean it's the correct amount for you to consume. If they did, then it would mean I would need to eat the same amount of food as my father, who is much taller and more muscular than I am. That doesn't make sense, does it?

The most important thing is listening to our bodies and knowing when they may need more or less than the recommended serving. However, serving sizes are definitely a good starting place. Sometimes, like in the case of ice cream, they may seem a little unrealistic. If you actually know how much ½ cup is, it's probably a lot smaller than the amount you usually put in your bowl. To give you a visual, a ½ cup is about the size of one cupped hand.

Unfortunately, Mary didn't know how much a ½ cup was, and she didn't have serving utensils on hand. Using her prior knowledge of what one serving of ice cream usually looks like, she scooped some into a bowl (and yes- this bowl was large like the bowls in most of our cabinets). Mary was excited because she guesstimated what seemed like ½ a cup. The Oreo Cookies & Cream flavor tasted heavenly to Mary. She was so happy that she was indulging in what her body was craving, while remaining aware of the portion. That seemed like the dream to her. The problem was, Mary didn't really know what ½ a cup looked like. Her bowl was filled with three cupped hand-sized scoops of ice cream. That means that she actually served herself 1½ cups. That's three times the recommended serving. It totals 390 calories and 42 grams of sugar.

It's no wonder that she felt sick soon after she finished her ice cream. She was so frustrated! She tried so hard to do everything right, yet somehow she was still overeating and not just by a few bites. Mary is not alone. It is extremely difficult for our brains to estimate serving sizes. To help illustrate this concept, we can use the vertical line illusion. Take a look at the lines below. Which is longer?

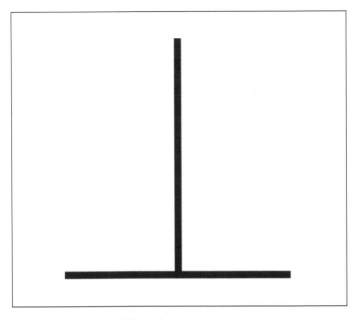

You may automatically think vertical, as I did. If you say that you thought they were the same length, you're right (and possibly a genius for catching that). Look one more time at the lines above, then look down to the same lines below, this time paired with a ruler. Our brains tend to overestimate the height of objects. You can see how this makes estimating serving sizes impossible. No matter how many times I look at those two lines with full awareness that they are the same length, I always see the vertical line as longer.

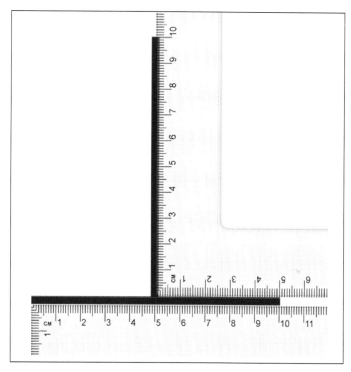

Credit: Wikipedia Commons—Public Domain

This means that even if Mary had known that ½ a cup was about the size of a tennis ball, she probably still would have served herself too much ice cream.

Unfortunately, Mary did not CUSP it. But, it wasn't when she chose to eat ice cream that she abandoned the method; it was when she did not listen to her body's signal of satisfaction. See that's the amazing thing about CUSP. It doesn't say you can't have ice cream!

In fact, it tells you that you should have ice cream if you're craving it. You should always **concentrate** on what your body is in the mood for. Mary can **understand** the nutritional value of her ice cream (U). She knows ice cream is filled with dairy (which our bodies need). Other than that, she knows it's a lot of "empty calories." But, those empty calories will prevent Mary from overeating in the future. This is one of the main reasons CUSP is a successful technique.

Mary didn't necessarily **supplement** (S) her ice cream with any other nutrients. It's not something that is going to make or break her health because as long as she remembers **portion** (P), Mary will be limiting how many of those "empty calories" she actually consumes. But that's not what happened. Mary didn't follow the most critical step. She failed to portion correctly. But the worst part is that she tried.

Who likes trying at something and still failing? No one! But Mary doesn't have to fail. She just needs a little help from the CUSP method.

The amazing thing about the CUSP method is that you cannot fail at it. CUSP doesn't say, "If you don't portion exactly according to guidelines you are no longer healthy." Instead, CUSP says, "How did you feel after eating that large bowl of ice cream? Uncomfortably full? Sluggish? Next time, listen to how you are feeling while you are eating the ice cream, and your body's internal cues will help you portion. By doing this, even those times when you serve yourself (or are served) a few more scoops than you need, your body will tell you when you have eaten enough to feel satisfied."

That being said, the best way to estimate a serving size is not to estimate at all. You can eat more or less than serving size based on how you feel and what your body wants and needs. However, when you are trying to have an idea of how much is generally recommended of a certain food, measuring can help. It's unrealistic to assume everyone will have all sorts of serving measurements available at all times, but stocking our kitchens with a few inexpensive plastic serving size guides can be a quick and easy fix for serving estimation. Instead of wondering whether or not you portioned a healthy size, know you did.

The difficulty in estimating servings is not something that only applies to college students. However, there is one thing about Mary and her millennial classmates that may be different from the general population. As you now know, portions have seen unprecedented growth in the past 60-70 years. Much of this growth, however, was at the time when millennials were either not yet born or were too young to remember. Although it is true that portions have grown during the lifetime of millennials, the rate at which they have grown is smaller than it was for generations before, like the silent generation or the baby boomers.

My theory is that millennials, like Mary, find estimating serving sizes even more difficult because they lack a frame of reference. When I ask my grandmother about portion increases, she can remember the blueberry muffins she used to eat were a lot smaller than those sold today. And she's right. Blueberry muffins have grown from about 1.5 ounces in 1950 to 5 ounces today. But what about Mary? She may be able to remember a few small increases since her childhood, but sadly, she and her classmates were born into a society already filled with over-sized portions. Without a frame of reference, a task that is normally extremely challenging for most human beings becomes nearly impossible for millennials.

The good news is that Mary is not doomed. The bad news is that estimating serving sizes takes time, practice and most importantly, actual measuring tools. In settings where access to these tools is impractical, visual estimations can at least help. The table below is a guide that can help during those times of need (because luckily we never forget our hands the way we forget our keys and wallets).

Hand Guideline	Serving Size	Food Example
Palm of your Hand	3-4 Ounces	Meat, Fish & Poultry
Two Cupped Hands	1 Ounce	Chips, Crackers & Pretzels
Fist	1 Cup	Fruits, Vegetables, Milk, Soup & Cereal
One Cupped Hand	½ Cup	Pasta, Rice, Beans & Ice Cream
Thumb	1-2 Tablespoons	Peanut Butter, Hard Cheeses & Salad Dressings
Thumbnail	1 Teaspoon	Butters, Oils & Mayonnaise

© Jaclyn DiGregorio 2017

* * *

CHANGES YOU CAN MAKE IN YOUR LIFE TODAY:

- Use recommended serving size as a place to start, but not as a place to finish
  - Always listen to your body's hunger cues
- Purchase inexpensive serving measurement utensils and use them in your kitchen at home
- When you're not at home, use your hands to estimate serving size
  - Palm = 3-4 ounces
  - Two cupped hands = 1 ounce
  - Fist = 1 cup

- One cupped hand = ½ cup
- Thumb = 1-2 tablespoons
- Thumbnail = 1 teaspoon
- If none of the hand estimations apply to what you're attempting to estimate and you're not home... fear not!
  - Remember the vertical line illusion and aim to underestimate the height of a serving. This will make up for the natural overestimation your brain will make for the height of a serving

PART 2 ·

CONCENTRATE

Concentrating on what your body is in the mood for is absolutely central to your long-term health and weight maintenance. Unfortunately, most people fail right here, at the first step.

We all know someone who successfully lost a great deal of weight but simply could not keep it off. You may even be this person yourself.

Our human nature frequently kicks in when someone tries to tell us we can't do something. We have a natural unquenchable thirst to prove that person wrong. We are free. We CAN do anything we want. This, of course, includes what we eat. When we try to tell ourselves that we "can't" have certain foods, our bodies tense up. They become angry. They let our minds control them for a short period and then they backfire. They send intense cravings to our minds for all those foods we forbid ourselves from eating. We may be able to fight these cravings for another short period, but eventually our bodies win out.

Dr. Pauline Wallin explains this idea through the psychological concept of heightened attention. She states, "When something is hard to get (or forbidden), you immediately pay more attention to it. Notice that when you are on a restricted diet, you sometimes get too focused on what you 'can't' eat. This heightened attention — which can escalate into obsession — makes the forbidden food seem very important."

It's a losing battle that's not worth fighting. And, the worst part is, we are not happy or healthy.

It's time to stop fighting with our bodies and instead nurture them with what they need. It's time to follow CUSP and it all starts with the first step—concentrate.

CHAPTER 4

FREEDOM OF CHOICE

IN THIS CHAPTER YOU WILL LEARN:

- How children's lack of choice in what they eat in their homes often translates to a lack of habit formation in terms of their own eating patterns
- The disastrous effects of not having established eating habits before entering college
- Why keeping certain foods "off-limits" in your home will often result in the opposite of the desired effect as soon as children get their hands on said foods for the first time

* * *

17-year-old Claire Brown was upstairs in her room doing homework when she heard her mom yell, "Claire…James… dinner!" She and her brother were used to this routine. Her mother cooked delicious, healthy meals for her family every day. Claire ran to the table to see what was on the menu for today. It was whole-wheat pasta with brussels sprouts, broc-coli, carrots, and grilled chicken. Yummy! Claire loved all of the meals her mom prepared. She never had to worry about what she would eat for dinner, because she knew her mother would whip up something delicious.

Mrs. Brown is what Dr. Wansink refers to as the "nutritional gatekeeper." This person purchases and prepares most of the meals in a household. As the nutritional gatekeeper, Mrs. Brown influences about 70% of what Claire, James, and her husband eat. Because Mrs. Brown encourages her family to eat healthy and balanced meals, she was not too concerned about Claire's eating habits when she went off to college. Boy, was Mrs. Brown shocked to see that Claire had gained five pounds when she came home for Thanksgiving.

If Claire had been taught to eat healthy since she was a child, what happened when she arrived at college? The problem with households like the Brown's, is that children don't form their own habits. Claire sat at the kitchen table and ate whatever her mother prepared for her. She enjoyed the healthy meals, but she never had the freedom to choose what she was having. Sometimes Mrs. Brown would request an opinion of what Claire or James was in the mood for, but their choices were limited to the typical meals their mother cooked.

Many college students come from households like Claire's. Even if every meal isn't as healthy as Mrs. Brown's, many parents at minimum serve a balanced meal consisting of a starch, a protein and a vegetable. Registered Dietitian Robyn Filpse explained to me that students find it most difficult to replicate healthy habits because college is often the first time they actually have to make the choice of what to eat for themselves. Children and teenagers may choose how much of each food group to put on their plate, but their choices are limited to whatever is on their table.

As a result, most college freshmen have not yet formed their own eating habits upon arrival. They have always eaten what was in front of them and had very little choice in the matter. When the time comes for students to actually make those decisions themselves, most just don't know what to choose.

Students like Claire were never taught the first step of the CUSP method, and that's where it all begins—concentrate on what your body is in the mood for. Claire rarely if ever had the opportunity to truly concentrate on what her body was in the mood for and chose to eat that food. Therefore, when Claire had no idea what to fill her plate with, of course her meal wasn't balanced and of course portions were not even considered. Without balance and awareness of portions, it's no wonder Claire struggled with her weight.

Claire's weight gain was also influenced by an exertion of autonomy against her parents. This is extremely common as freshman experience newfound freedoms in not only what they eat and drink, but also where they go, who they go with, and when they come home (or don't come home). Especially coming from a household like the Brown's, Claire wanted to eat everything that she was never allowed to eat in the past.

Mrs. Brown rarely, if ever, kept dessert in the house, so that was Claire's main go-to. There was a large selection of cookies, brownies, and ice cream at her cafeteria's dessert bar. This was available for students during every meal, even breakfast! Maybe if dessert was more readily available to Claire during her childhood, she would not have rebelled and overindulged as soon as she was on her own for the first time. It's wonderful that Mrs. Brown encourages her family to eat healthy, but too much restriction during childhood can lead to an abuse of freedom later in life.

It's the same concept as the restriction on allowing teenagers to stay out late. If a high school boy was given a curfew of 9 p.m. on weekends, as soon as he arrives at college, I can almost guarantee you that he will be staying out all night long in rebellion of that curfew. On the contrary, if his curfew was midnight, staying out until 1 or 2 a.m. isn't such a big deal anymore. This does not mean that Mrs. Brown should have served sugary desserts with every single meal, but keeping something sweet in the house for the times her children were craving a treat would have lessened the future over-consumption.

* * *

CHANGES YOU CAN MAKE IN YOUR LIFE TODAY:

- Allow your children (pre-college) to choose meals you serve in your home
  - This teaches them how to create a balanced meal with healthy portion sizes so they already have these habits formed when they enter college
- Don't keep foods "off-limits" in your home
  - Encourage your children to listen to what their bodies are craving
  - Purchase any meals, treats, or snacks your family requests
  - Teach your family how to portion these meals, treats and snacks so they can enjoy them and not worry about over-eating them

CHAPTER 5

MORE CHOICES, MORE CALORIES

IN THIS CHAPTER YOU WILL LEARN:

- How the number of food choices influences how much you will eat
- How to approach the almost infinite choices in an all-you-can eat cafeteria
- How to alter meals in your own home to help with preventing overeating

* * *

Like most students their first time inside a college cafeteria, Jake was completely overwhelmed by the numerous food choices surrounding him. Everything looked and smelled absolutely delicious. So, he decided that he would have no choice but to try everything. If he only tried a small amount of each food he wanted, he thought that he wouldn't overeat. Before Jake knew it, his plate was overfull. He had no space for the remaining foods he wanted to try. Not wanting to eat two plates of food, Jake settled for the one very stuffed plate and piled on the remaining must haves as he finished browsing the cafeteria. It was clear to him that his initial plan of only tasting small amounts of each option was still resulting in a substantial amount of food.

With so many choices, portioning becomes a very difficult task. Even if we only fill our plate with a little of everything, we can see that our plate will still be overfull. Remember to keep it simple and CUSP it. Fill your plate with the foods you're in the mood for and make sure the meal is balanced. When following CUSP, we know that portioning is the most important part. So make portioning as easy as possible for yourself. Limit your own choices, even in an environment where there are so many.

Dr. Susan Racette holds a PhD in human nutrition and nutritional biology. She described this human tendency to me. Racette said, "Choices alone have a big influence on how much people eat. The more choices a person has, the more a person will eat." Because college cafeterias offer virtually unlimited choices, it becomes very difficult for students not to overeat. At home, it's much easier to limit choices. All you have to do is cook less, and who would complain about that? Instead of cooking both chicken and steak as the protein of your meal, only cook one. Those consuming the meal will naturally eat less, due to the limitation on choice.

Unfortunately, for Jake, we cannot ask the chefs in college cafeterias to cook less variety of foods. A large variety is necessary when serving thousands of students for allergy, preference and simply to accommodate large numbers. By concentrating on what his body is in the mood for, Jake can choose a single food option that will satisfy him. That way, he will eliminate the additional calories that come with additional choices. With multiple floors each filled with a plethora of food stations, Jake can decide to have make-your-own tacos one day and make-your-own rice bowl the next.

The same goes for your company's cafeteria and that all you-can-eat restaurant at which your family dines. Make one choice of what you want and stick to it. Be your own limiter of choice to minimize mindless overeating. Whether it be at home or in a cafeteria, don't fall victim to wanting "just a little piece" of eight different foods. Aiming to have only one protein and one starch can be a great way to do this. (Notice I didn't say only one veggie, because most people don't have problems with eating too many veggies—so go for as many as you'd like—but don't eat too large of a portion, of course.) As overwhelming as a multi-story cafeteria filled with food can be, if Jake focuses on eating a single balanced meal that he's in the mood for, he will be on track to the happy, healthy lifestyle we all strive to enjoy.

* * *

CHANGES YOU CAN MAKE IN YOUR LIFE TODAY:

- In a college dining hall, corporate cafeteria or buffet restaurant, choose only one protein and one starch to put on your plate
  - Choose your favorite of each; you can enjoy a meal you love while eating healthy portions
- When cooking a meal, only serve one protein and one starch to encourage not overeating these food groups
  - Ex: Choose either potatoes or pasta for the starch of the meal, don't even offer both because if you do, people will put both on their plates and almost definitely fill more than ¼ of their plate with starch
  - By limiting choice, you are encouraging your family to eat smaller portions, which is the secret weapon
  - Consider cooking more than one vegetable (or offering cooked vegetables and salad) to encourage more consumption of these superfoods

CHAPTER 6

THE TIME-CONSUMPTION CORRELATION

IN THIS CHAPTER YOU WILL LEARN:

- How time spent in an eating area (applies to college dining halls, corporate cafeterias, and your kitchen at home) influences how much you eat
- Why finding a "hang-out spot" other than the cafeteria or kitchen may be beneficial
- How we can manage portions simply by limiting the amount of time we spend in an eating area (like cafeteria or kitchen)

* * *

Alex glanced down at her watch and was in disbelief that

three hours had already passed. She had arrived at the dining hall with her roommates around 5:00 that evening. About an hour before she left her dorm, Alex decided that she was too hungry to wait to eat. She grabbed a banana with peanut butter and some crackers to satisfy her hunger. She was already full from her snack and knew that she wouldn't be hungry for a meal until at least a few more hours passed. Nonetheless, the cafeteria was the social utopia of the freshman community, and Alex couldn't miss out on that.

Every time a new group of friends joined, Alex made herself an additional plate of food. Two hours and three plates later, Alex walked out of the cafeteria feeling the way most freshman did after each meal, uncomfortably full. By continuing to eat past the point of being full, Alex was not concentrating on what her body was in the mood for. If your body is no longer hungry, stop eating. Always concentrate on your internal hunger cues.

Alex may not have realized it, but the more time she spent in the dining hall, the more food she put in front of herself. I call this the time-consumption correlation. More time in the cafeteria = more food consumed. The same concept applies to your kitchen. The more time spent at the kitchen table or just sitting in the kitchen relaxing, the more likely you are to eat, even when you're not hungry. The obvious way to alleviate the effects of the time-consumption correlation is to minimize your time in the dining area (i.e. the college cafeteria or your kitchen at home).

Yet again, by spending more time in an eating area, like the dining hall or your kitchen, you're making living that healthy, happy and balanced life extremely difficult, when in reality it's quite simple. By simply CUSPing it, you can choose to eat whatever you're in the mood for and create a balanced meal, but unless you portion (and that means don't go back up for seconds and thirds), you're probably doing yourself more harm than good. Make portioning easy for yourself by limiting the time you spend in the dining hall or your kitchen.

One way for college students to do this is to plan meals between other commitments. For example, if Alex were to go to the dining hall when she finished class at 6:00 and had to be at a group project meeting by 7:30, she wouldn't have a choice but to leave the dining hall by 7:15. She would likely only spend an hour eating dinner, which is more than enough time. Alex should try to eat slowly; remember it takes about 20 minutes for hormone signals to let our brains know that we are full.

As for your kitchen at home, it's best to not use it as a relaxation spot. This can be very tempting for those who have TVs in their kitchens. Watch TV in a different room, and in general try not to linger too long after finishing a meal. If you do linger because you are enjoying time with family and friends, try to be more aware of how much additional food you are putting on your plate simply because you are still sitting at the table. Only go back for seconds if you are truly still hungry and your body has already had 20 minutes to register fullness.

* * *

CHANGES YOU CAN MAKE IN YOUR LIFE TODAY:

- Limit the time you spend in a dining hall all-you-can-eat buffet
  - Force deadlines by scheduling other places you need to be right after, so you can't stay longer than planned
- Stop eating when you are no longer hungry
- Don't relax in your kitchen
  - Move the TV into a different room
  - If you're spending hours chatting with your family or friends at the table after a meal, suggest you take the conversation into another room where everyone will be more comfortable anyway
- Always wait 20 minutes after finishing your meal before grabbing seconds to be sure you are still hungry (I know you have heard this before, but I also know you probably don't always follow this rule and may need a reminder)

CHAPTER 7

FINANCIAL MOTIVATORS OF A CAFETERIA

IN THIS CHAPTER YOU WILL LEARN:

- How one all-you-can-eat price impacts calorie consumption (with complete disregard for portions)
- How to both financially and nutritiously get the most out of your meal plan (yes, it's possible)
- How to approach an all-you-can eat buffet or corporate cafeteria

* * *

When Lauren was a freshman in college, her parents wanted to be sure she never had to worry about where she was going to eat. They chose the largest (and most expensive) meal plan for their daughter, which included three meals per day. Lauren felt very grateful. She made a conscious effort to "get her parents' money's worth" every time she swiped into the cafeteria by making sure she felt full every time she left. She would never waste a meal swipe on a small salad.

Lauren's best friend, Kara, also followed Lauren's footsteps in eating as much as she could every time she used a meal swipe. Kara's thought process, however, was much different from Lauren's. Kara didn't feel guilty that her parents had also chosen the most expensive meal plan, instead she felt very happy. FREE MEALS! It was basically like free money. Kara could eat as much as she wanted and not have to spend a penny. What a steal. Lauren and Kara both are examples of students who attempt to maximize their calories per dollar. This is an extremely common behavioral norm among college students, whether or not most are even aware of it.

Professor David Levitsky, who teaches Nutrition and Psychology at Cornell University, described to me his theory that because of fixed dining fees, students naturally attempt to maximize their calories per dollar in order to get the most out of their dining plan. They aim to put as much on their plates as possible, and throw away what they don't eat, creating potential issues such as food waste (again we see this problem!!!). There is nothing inherently wrong with them wanting to eat enough cafeteria food so that their parents' investment (or for some students, their personal investment) in their meal plan becomes worth it. As college expenses continue to grow, I can't imagine students wanting anything else.

How can students follow the CUSP method in an environment where they need to eat as much as possible to really get their "money's worth?" Sure, they can choose what to eat based on their cravings, and sure they can also craft a balanced meal. But, how is it possible to portion while trying to eat as much as they can? It's not. But, you're in luck. I have found a solution to both maximize calories per dollar AND follow CUSP.

It is possible for Lauren and Kara to still make the most of their meal plans, while not overeating each time they use a meal swipe. It's called taking food to-go. Many colleges even provide containers for students to take their left overs (so if this is the case, fill up). In colleges that do not provide this, students can usually bring their own Tupperware and grab some food for a later day. If, however, you do attend a university that has strict food policies, you can always grab fruit and pre-wrapped food and place it right in your backpack.

This mindset of wanting to "get your money's worth" of something, which Lauren and Kara represent, is not out of the ordinary. It's actually characteristic of how the average person thinks. In fact, Levitsky explained, "The number one reason that people go back to restaurants is that they think they are getting the maximum amount of food for their dollar." Therefore, as you can imagine, this phenomenon is not limited solely to college dining halls. The same happens in your favorite all-you-can-eat Chinese buffets and Brazilian steakhouses and even those all-you-can-eat salad bars.

Unfortunately, all-you-can-eat buffet restaurants or corporate cafeterias do not offer to-go containers. The best thing you can do for yourself if you are going to an all-you-can-eat buffet for a meal is to be aware of the financial motivators. Think about how much money you are spending and how much you would like to eat. If you truly want to maximize your calories per dollar and have an achy belly after you finish your meal, go for it. My argument is not that doing this would be a bad thing (although obviously, we both know it's not the best decision in terms of your health), the problem is more that we are not aware of this motivator. I, personally, despise feeling sick after overeating, and even at a buffet, I don't want to feel this way.

Outside the setting of a dining hall, you at least have the choice of whether or not you want to go to a buffet for dinner. If you're concerned about this dilemma of "getting the bang for your buck" but also feeling uncomfortably full after eating so much, maybe just consider going somewhere else. However, for Lauren and Kara, their meal swipes are prepaid, so they do not have the luxury of choosing to eat elsewhere.

Additionally, as freshmen, these prepaid meal plans are required at the majority of colleges. The best that students like Lauren and Kara can do is be aware of this motivator and aim to stop eating when full and take leftovers to go for another meal later in the day or the week. By concentrating on what their bodies are in the mood for, the girls can eat based on their cravings and hunger cues, not financial motivators. Anything their bodies are not in the mood for while they are in the dining hall can be carried out for later.

* * *

CHANGES YOU CAN MAKE IN YOUR LIFE TODAY:

- Carefully portion the meal that you eat in the dining hall as you would any meal according to CUSP
  - Take extra food in to-go containers if your college or university allows it
- Consider the impact an all-you-can-eat price will have on how much you eat (and how over-sized your portions will be)
  - Maybe forgo the buffet and instead choose a restaurant where you pay based on what you order
    - Often the less you order, the less you spend—you can still get your "money's worth" at your average restaurant
- Always concentrate on cravings and hunger cues to guide how much you eat, even in an unlimited setting

PART 3

UNDERSTAND

You know those complicated subjects that have books written about them solely to simplify the dense material. They're usually called something like, "_____ For Dummies."

CUSP doesn't need something like this because it is already so easy to understand.

That's how we arrive at step 2—Understand. CUSP doesn't require extensive nutrition knowledge or memorization of guidelines. It simply requires you to understand what food groups make up the meal you are about to eat. And to make it even easier, you only have to focus on fruits, veggies, protein, and starch.

Anyone can break down their meal into four simple food groups. If you need a little help here, just remember that most meats, dairy products, beans, eggs, fishes, nuts and nut butters are high in protein. And, most grains, pastas, potatoes, breads, and cereals are high in starch.

I am confident that you can figure out which foods are fruits and vegetables. And for those tricky ones like tomatoes or avocados, don't worry. You don't even have to distinguish between which are fruits and which are veggies because they all go into the one category in the CUSP method.

CHAPTER 8

THE DISAPPEARANCE OF SPORTS

IN THIS CHAPTER YOU WILL LEARN:

- The importance of maintaining the same exercise levels students had in high school during college
- How to transition from a structured sport to structuring your own workouts
- Seamless ways to add extra exercise into your schedule
- The important ways CUSP applies to exercise
- How to approach eating pre-and post-working out

* * *

In high school, John was a three-sport varsity athlete. He had practice almost every single day after school and his summers consisted of extra leagues and tournaments. John had been playing sports for as long as he could remember, and he was quite talented. For a combination of reasons, John decided not to play a varsity sport in college. The schools he was offered to play at were not the same universities that had the best-suited academic programs for his needs, and he knew that he wanted to shift his focus onto his studies and future career. This decision by no means meant that John would stop playing sports. He still plays pick-up games with his friends, on summer league teams and on club teams in college.

John was very content with his decision not to play a varsity sports in college. Club sports fit perfectly into his schedule without too much stress. The only thing that John didn't consider is how much a sudden drop in his levels of exercise would impact his strong, muscular physique. He quickly began to notice that his fitness capabilities were declining, like when he was short of breath during a soccer game or lost an arm wrestling match to his dad for the first time since 9th grade. From that point on, John wanted to be sure that he exercised every day or at least most days to maintain his high fitness goals.

At first, John's problem was finding time for the gym. It's a big adjustment going from a very regimented schedule that was created by a coach, to having to make up a schedule yourself. He decided to go to the gym at the same time every day, as if it were a sports practice. This solved his first problem, but he soon had another in front of him. What should he actually do at the gym?

John was only used to having very structured workouts. Yes, he lifted weights, used machines, did cardio etc., but his days in the gym consisted of him following a packet of exercises. He was instructed by his coaches on which machines to use, how much weight to put on them and how many reps to do. John replicated some of these workouts and eventually found a routine he enjoyed. That being said, the transition from playing sports 7 days a week to a few times a week was not the easiest for his body or for his new schedule.

John is like many college freshmen. The NCAA reports that, on average, only about 6% of high school athletes continue their career into college with a varsity sport. In the same way that many 18-year-olds have not formed eating habits if they rarely made their own decisions on what to eat, many of these same students have not formed exercise habits because they rarely made their own decisions about when and how to work out. This can be even worse for students who did not play sports in high school. For some, their only exercise may have come from PE class. A lack of structured exercise decreases the physical activeness of students on college campuses.

It perhaps goes without saying that exercise is extremely

important. In addition to the endless health benefits, there are many psychological benefits as well. Endorphins are real, and if you haven't experienced them within the past three days, go for a walk, run, bike ride, anything… just do something active! For students like John, going to the gym isn't the only way to fit exercise into your day. Most college campuses require a great deal of walking. Ridesharing apps have made students extremely lazy. I know it might be cold and raining outside, but if you have to go two blocks to a friend's house, get some extra steps in and save a few dollars. Walking more often can be a great way to supplement your day with extra exercise.

Think CUSP and apply it to exercise. Concentrate on what you are in the mood for. Do you want to do yoga, go for a swim, or do some other form of exercise? The same way you can choose any food you are in the mood for, you can choose any exercise you are in the mood for. It is most important just to get out there and do something.

Understanding is also critical in exercise. What do you want to accomplish? What are your goals? Write them down. Briefly research what types of exercise can help you achieve those goals. If you want to run a half marathon, check out some training guides and see how many miles you should be running each week to make that goal a reality. If you want to grow certain muscle groups, understand which exercises will have the best impact on those muscles.

And continue applying CUSP to your pre- and post-work out meals.

A big problem with exercise is that afterwards people often eat more calories than they burned because they feel they've "earned it." Try not to alter your eating routine on the days you've exercised versus days you haven't. Of course, as CUSP encourages, listen to your body. If you're hungrier and need more protein or carbs after a very intensive workout, feed your body those foods. But don't forget your veggies and don't forget your portions. It always comes back to balance and of course portions.

There are many easy ways that don't require a gym membership to implement additional exercise in your daily routine. If your grocery store is less than a mile away, try to walk there. Carrying your groceries back home is the ultimate workout (and helps you save money because you will only buy what you can carry). If this seems a little too extreme for your lifestyle, try parking in a spot that is further away from the entrance. Those extra steps going across the parking lot will add up. Tracking steps with a smartwatch or app can be very rewarding.

Don't let a change in routine impact the amount of time you schedule for exercise. Although not playing sports in college can make for a big change in physical activity, it also provides an opportunity to discover new forms of exercise. For all the grandparents reading this, you're never too old to fall in love with a new form of exercise. Your body will (hopefully) thank you with many additional years of life.

* * *

CHANGES YOU CAN MAKE IN YOUR LIFE TODAY:

- If you're having trouble making daily exercise part of your routine, try incorporating it into your schedule at the same time every day
- Just go out and do something active!! Today, tomorrow and the next day
    - Try walking to the grocery store and carrying your groceries home if it's not too far
    - Try parking your car farther away every time you run an errand
    - Opt for walking instead of using Uber or Lyft when heading to a friend's house or restaurant nearby
    - Try a new form of exercise you've yet to try—you just may fall in love with it
    - Aim to walk 10,000 steps per day
        - And track them—most smartphones automatically track them anyway, so you don't have to invest in a smartwatch or other wearable technology unless you want to

- - Don't let the cold stop you from hitting your step goal daily; walk circles inside your house if you have to
- Write down your exercise goals
  - Structure your workouts in a way that can help make those goals a reality
- Aim to eat basically the same (following the CUSP method) on days you exercise and days you don't
  - If you're following CUSP correctly, you may notice when concentrating that you are hungrier after a workout, of course listen to your body and fuel it with the recovery it needs

CHAPTER 9

THE FOOD-CENTRIC CULTURE WE LIVE IN

———

IN THIS CHAPTER YOU WILL LEARN:

- How our food-centric culture impacts our eating habits
- What to order when "grabbing lunch" with a friend
- Why sometimes we should appreciate our food-centric culture
- How to have your pie and eat it too
- Finding balance among those things that play both our devils and our angels

* * *

Thanksgiving has always been Julie's favorite holiday. She enjoys spending time with her family, expressing gratitude to her loved ones, and of course eating turkey, potatoes, and lots of pie. Ever since she has been away at college, Thanksgiving has become even more meaningful for Julie. It is the first weekend of the school year that she is able to fly home and catch up with her parents, siblings, aunts, uncles, cousins, grandparents and close friends from high school. During the celebrations, Julie often eats more than she intends. She is easily swept away into deep conversations with family members and mindlessly eats all that is in front of her. And we all know that on Thanksgiving, there is rarely a shortage of food in front of us.

No big deal though! Who cares if we overeat on Thanksgiving… it's only one day a year, right? If Thanksgiving was the only day of the year that Americans overate, the average American would probably weigh about 26 pounds less. But of course it's not. Food surrounds virtually everything we do. During every holiday, the two central components are family and food. There is always a reason to celebrate. It's constantly someone's birthday, graduation, engagement, wedding, retirement, baby shower… you name it. There will be a party and there will be food, and don't forget the dessert.

This is even more prevalent in the college environment. Due to students' constantly busy schedules packed with classes, projects, clubs and activities, volunteer work, internships, jobs and attempting to sleep, they have limited opportunity socialize with friends outside of these commitments. If they do, it's probably while drinking on a Saturday night and they likely didn't have a chance to fit in a real conversation at a loud party or bar.

This is where food comes in. The easiest way to see a friend and catch up is over a meal. Whether we like to admit it or not, we need to eat and not just a snack between commitments. Consuming protein bars for every meal will quickly remind your body that it needs nutrients to function properly. Snacks and bars don't cut it. So, students often turn to "grabbing lunch" as a 30-60 minute break to spend quality time with friends. This habit is just another environmental factor of the college lifestyle that makes maintaining a healthy lifestyle seem almost impossible.

Many of us love to eat out. And "grabbing lunch" with a friend continues much beyond college. As long as you always CUSP it when eating out, you'll enjoy a meal you love, fuel your body with balanced nutrition, and stop yourself from overeating by portioning.

Let's also take this time to note how amazing food is for all of the above reasons. Food brings people together. Some of my favorite conversations I've shared with family and friends have been sitting around the dinner table eating a big bowl of pasta (or insert some other yummy starch). I'm sure you can say the same. I would not trade those dinners or the cold winter nights I spent baking (and of course devouring) chocolate chip cookies with my mom and sisters for anything.

Some nutritionists believe that the one or two additional pounds a year that result from these meaningful dinners and desserts are worth every extra calorie. I would agree in the sense that it is worth it to enjoy those foods and moments, but I disagree that indulging in them necessarily leads to weight gain. Like everything else in life, nutrition is about balance. Eat a cookie when you bake them, just don't eat five. (But it's still okay if you do eat five. Listen to the way your body feels after eating five cookies and most likely, you will choose to eat only one cookie next time. When you choose one cookie, again listen to how your body feels. I can tell you from experience, it will probably be happy and satisfied. When you remember those feelings, choosing to eat one cookie becomes second nature.)

I am confident that if you stop overeating (this means rarely if ever feeling "overly full" again in your life) and eat until you are satisfied and focus on balance, those extra pounds won't exist. And you can still have the cookies! I know by this point you know that the CUSP method helps you do just that. Eat the cookies when you are in the mood, as long as you don't eat too many. If you concentrate on the signals your body sends, you will know when you're full and stop eating at that point.

This aside, our food-centric culture makes it difficult to behave in this way. It's not as easy as it sounds when enjoying appetizers at a friend's party to say to yourself, "I've already had enough cheese and crackers. I'm no longer hungry, so I will immediately walk away from this table and let the thought of eating any more leave my mind". If you do think like that, you're probably a superhuman (or some sort of robot—who knows with today's technology). So what can we do? Food is our angel and our devil. It can be the home of some of our favorite memories and at the same time some of our worst overeating and self-loathing experiences.

Many things in life can play as our angel and our devil simultaneously. A job that you like for the money it provides your family with but hate the long hours. A relationship that you love for the happiness it brings you but hate for the lack of attention and respect you receive. Any form of addiction: drugs, alcohol, even caffeine creates this same love-hate relationship.

We all have our own devils and angels, and unfortunately at times and fortunately at other times, food is included in this list. All we can do is appreciate the angel and be conscious of the devil. For Julie, she should recognize how food plays such a special role in her Thanksgiving. She can appreciate and savor every bite she takes and understand that her meal is central to her family's celebration. At the same time, Julie should remember that if she eats three slices of pie and then feels uncomfortably full, she will ruin this time with family that she treasures so much. By following CUSP and portioning her pie into one slice instead of three, Julie can truly enjoy her pie along with her company, without having to jump on a post-Thanksgiving diet the next morning.

The great thing about most holidays is that the foods offered are balanced. Most thanksgiving meals consist of: turkey (protein), white or sweet potatoes (starch), green beans or carrots (veggies) and cranberries (fruit). This makes the process of understanding which food groups we are eating on those big holidays relatively simple.

My mother always told me to accept people for who they are. This means appreciating the good they bring to your life and being aware of the bad. Julie's meal is the same. By appreciating the good and being aware of the bad, Julie can set a great example for all of us to live happy and balanced lives in our food-centric culture.

* * *

CHANGES YOU CAN MAKE IN YOUR LIFE TODAY:

- Always CUSP it when you are eating out (or eating anywhere for that matter)

- Be that person who enjoys baking holiday cookies with family, but also knows not to eat six cookies.
  - Indulging in cravings + portioning = you really can have it all
- Eat the pie on Thanksgiving, the cake on your son's birthday, and the ice cream at your mom's retirement party—but portion yourself one slice, not three
- Identify three things in your life right now that play as both your devil and angel (food can be one of them)
  - Think about ways you can appreciate the good more—and do those
  - Think about ways you can be more aware of the bad—and do those as well

CHAPTER 10

THE DANGERS OF EMOTIONAL EATING

———

IN THIS CHAPTER YOU WILL LEARN:

- Why humans eat emotionally
- When eating emotionally becomes dangerous
- How to handle emotional cravings in a healthy way
- Other ways (besides food) through which we can express our emotions
- How to distinguish between physical hunger and emotional hunger

* * *

Kyle was dreading his managerial accounting class with every bone in his body. The day had come that his professor was going to hand back the dreaded midterm that he had taken a few weeks ago. It was definitely the hardest test he had ever taken in his life. He knew that he did not do well. Kyle was praying that he would at least pass. Of course, his professor waited until the end of class to hand back the midterm. When Kyle caught sight of his grade, he immediately thought that it had to be a mistake. "An A-!!?" Amazing – he thought to himself. As he flipped through his test, Kyle realized that he had truly earned the A. He was so happy.

Kyle called his roommate Joe, who had been listening to him complain about his grades in this class throughout the semester. Joe suggested they go out and get ice cream to celebrate. He would have suggested drinks, but both of the boys had 8 a.m. classes in the morning, so ice cream sounded like the perfect option. The boys loaded up on chocolate syrup, sprinkles, and all kinds of candy on top. In that moment, Kyle could not have been happier. What a great way to celebrate his A.

Kyle is human. Humans eat emotionally. Therefore, yes, Kyle was victim to emotional eating the same way that you and I are as well. The alternative to this is eating emotionlessly. Do you live to eat or eat to live? If we truly ate to live, there would be no purpose for this book. There would be no subconscious motivators that influence how we eat, because we would solely eat exactly what our bodies needed and nothing more. But we don't. We live to eat. Food tastes delicious, and we naturally celebrate and grieve with food.

A common form of emotional eating is using food as a coping mechanism when things in life aren't going exactly the way a person wants. Your friend's boyfriend breaks up with her; you go buy her some cookie dough. Your boss gives you a bad performance review; you go home and order pizza for dinner. Often times, emotional eating leads to overeating followed by feelings of guilt. Registered Dietitian Rachael Hartley explains, "Feelings of guilt and shame not only affect digestion and how you metabolize food, but keep you trapped in the emotional eating cycle. When you feel guilty for emotionally eating, you'll continue to emotionally eat."

This cycle is dangerous because you start to give food power over yourself. Emotional eating is not intrinsically bad. If I have a great day and want to eat a cookie to celebrate, I should eat a cookie. Or, if I have a horrible day and want to eat a cookie to help cheer myself up, I should eat a cookie. There is nothing wrong with either of these situations, as long as I consciously make the choice and am aware that I am not hungry but instead am giving into an emotional craving. That's exactly what Kyle did. He recognized that he was eating this ice cream to celebrate his A. Go Kyle!

Having emotional cravings is in fact, totally normal. Better yet, it's encouraged by the CUSP method. The first step is to concentrate on what you are in the mood for. Sometimes, we are in the mood for lots of sugar or fried foods to help us cope with or celebrate an emotion. What makes CUSP really work is the method as a whole, not just one part. So C alone (concentrating on those cravings) isn't going to help us live healthy, happy, balanced lives.

We also have to understand the food groups of the ice cream, supplement it with missing groups, and most importantly portion. Kyle may admit that although his ice cream could use some more supplemental fruits and/or veggies, he chose not to add them. As long as he remembers the last step of CUSP (portion), I am not too worried. Kyle can understand that a healthy portion of ice cream contains dairy and fat that his body can use. And with a healthy portion, there is little room for damage.

On the other hand, if the only way we know how to deal with our emotions is through food, serious problems begin to develop. As a human being (and especially a 21 year-old female), I have many emotions that run through my head every few seconds. I would have to eat about 50 cookies a day to cope with all of my emotions (both positive and negative). And, no one would disagree that 50 cookies in one day would be very counterproductive to my health. Instead, I might eat one cookie, go for a run, write in my journal, read a book, hang with friends, listen to music, etc. to soothe my many feelings. This is a much healthier and more balanced way to cope with my emotions.

There are many times in life that we can be happy to make the choice to eat emotionally, like appreciating every bite of sweet cake on your wedding day or savoring all the flavors in your pasta the first time you visit Italy. It's important to be able to distinguish these moments so we can decide when we want to eat emotionally and when we don't. Food doesn't need to be a reward for us. But, it can be, when we want it to be.

It's important for us to be able to differentiate feelings of emotional hunger and feelings of physical hunger. Your hunger is emotionally driven when it comes on suddenly, is in the form of specific foods (often "comfort" foods high in sugar), results in you feeling uncomfortably full without satisfaction and leaves you with feelings of guilt or regret. You can probably recall a time (or two or three) that you've felt this way in the past.

One test that makes it easy to tell if you are physically hungry or not is called the broccoli test. Ask yourself, "am I so hungry right now that I would eat raw broccoli?" Most of us probably have a memory of a time that we have felt like this. For one reason or another, you skipped a meal or let too much time go by between meals. Your stomach physically aches and you would do just about anything to eat immediately. You would eat anything edible, even foods you strongly dislike.

That is what true physical hunger feels like (of course in an extreme case). If you are hungry, you would take the broccoli. If you're simply emotionally eating, like Kyle was with his ice cream, you would pass on the broccoli. (And, if you truly are a broccoli lover, pick a food to substitute in that phrase that you don't love as much).

Once you know whether you are physically hungry or just emotionally hungry, you can make your own decision to eat emotionally or not. If you have concluded that you are emotionally hungry and would like to eat anyway (again nothing wrong with this), try to pinpoint what is causing your emotional hunger. For example, tell yourself something like, "I know that I am not physically hungry, but I want a brownie anyway because I was pulled over for a speeding ticket on my way home from work today." The more you understand your motivation the better you can deal with it, not only with food, but with other coping mechanisms.

Just remember when dealing with emotional eating, like all forms of eating, it's about balance. If you do decide to go for your craving, eat mindfully. Taste and enjoy every single bite. By doing this, you are focusing on the pleasurable experience the food is giving you, and you are much less likely to continue eating when you are no longer experiencing pleasure - once you are full. By giving into your craving but eating in moderation, you can enjoy the food you emotionally wanted without feeling guilty afterwards, and you can help your body feel satisfied without feeling deprived.

If you want to avoid the emotional craving altogether, try to find other ways to mitigate whatever is bothering you. If you are lonely, call a friend or visit a neighbor. If you are bored, go for a walk or watch your favorite TV show. If you are celebrating, get a massage or manicure and pedicure. Find your own ways that do not include food both to deal with negative feelings and to reward yourself for positive feelings. But remember, emotional eating is okay, because we are humans. We are on this earth to enjoy our lives, not to restrict and control everything. Sometimes, we need to celebrate an achievement with ice cream just like Kyle (or cake, cookies AND ice cream for those really big achievements), and that's perfectly okay.

* * *

CHANGES YOU CAN MAKE IN YOUR LIFE TODAY:

- Each time you go to grab something to eat, pause and ask yourself if you're truly physically hungry or you're just emotionally hungry (symptoms below):

- Your hunger came on suddenly
- You're craving specific sugary foods
- You're currently celebrating a success or coping with a failure
  - Ask yourself, "Am I so hungry right now that I would eat raw broccoli?"
- Following the CUSP method, sometimes you will eat emotionally—don't fret
  - Focus on the portion size; keep the portions of foods you are emotionally craving small
  - Identify the source of your emotions, that way you can deal with it in other ways as well
- Try three new ways to deal with your emotions
  - Exercise
  - Visit a neighbor
  - Treat yourself to a massage or mani/pedi
  - Watch your favorite TV show
  - Take a nap

PART 4

SUPPLEMENT

One main point of the CUSP method is to help you become a healthier version of yourself through the creation and consumption of balanced meals. So far, with steps one and two, we have only been identifying our desires and their nutritional value. If we stop here, we will be far from healthy, and far from happy, because we won't feel right. Our bodies will be lacking essential nutrients. We will be groggy, unproductive and probably overweight.

So what's next? We must supplement our meals with the nutrients they are currently lacking, to create a balanced diet. When you follow step two of CUSP and recognize the major food groups you are craving, you also recognize what food groups are missing. These missing groups are the ones we must supplement our meal with. Always do your best to add the necessary foods to your meal so that it follows the following guidelines: ½ of the meal is fruits or veggies, ¼ of the meal is protein and ¼ of the meal is starch.

If you can learn this balance and how to apply it to nutrition, I guarantee you that it will transfer to other areas of your life. Even in the craziest of times, everything will feel just a little more in balance and a little more peaceful.

CHAPTER 11

UNHEALTHY HABITS ARE MORE CONTAGIOUS THAN THE FLU

——

IN THIS CHAPTER YOU WILL LEARN:

- How the unhealthy choices of one friend or family member can be detrimental to those around him or her
- How easily what we choose to eat is influenced by those around us
- How following the CUSP method can result in ordering the food you were craving but prevent you from feeling guilty afterward

＊＊＊

Samantha, a sophomore in college, felt that she generally ate healthy most of the time. She gained a few pounds when she began college last year, as most students do, but she shed them over the summer by being more cognizant of both what and how much she ate. There were times, however, when Samantha felt like she'd fallen back into all of her old unhealthy habits again. This happened almost every time she went out to eat or to the dining hall with friends. She recalled an example of a recent experience like this, "I was excited to go to this cool new restaurant that opened up near campus with friends. I wanted to try their salmon salad. I checked out the menu ahead of time to be sure I could find something that was healthy and that I would enjoy," Samantha explained.

"When my friends and I were sitting at our table looking over our menus, one of my roommates, Katie, said she was going to order a cheeseburger and french fries. As soon as she spoke, another one of my friends, Hannah, commented that a burger and fries sounded amazing, and she was going to order that as well. Before I knew it, all of the other girls were ordering cheeseburgers. How could I get a salad? A burger and fries can't be THAT bad for you if all of my friends are ordering it, right?"

Samantha used her friends' unhealthy choices to justify her own guilt-filled decision. Because everyone around her was ordering a 1000+ calorie meal, she didn't feel so bad about simply following their lead. It's like that voice inside of your head that's screaming, "I want pizza," but you are planning on ordering a salad. As soon as someone you're with goes for the pizza, the words fly out of your mouth before you've even processed that you're saying them. Before you know it, the pizza is in front of you.

We have all been in this situation before. If everyone at a party eats three pieces of cake, it doesn't seem as bad as if I were to eat three pieces of cake by myself. However, in reality, either way you are still eating three pieces of cake. It's much easier to be subconsciously manipulated into eating the three pieces when others around you are doing the same.

Unhealthy habits are certainly contagious. In a dining hall setting, where students are constantly eating with friends, the danger multiplies. Dr. Wansink studied how much of the food students serve themselves is influenced by what the person in front of them serves him or herself. He explained to me that, "44% of how much you eat at a dining hall is determined by what you serve yourself and this is determined by what the person in front of you served him or herself. This primarily occurs in females following females in line at the cafeteria." No surprise in that, ladies. Sadly, we all know how self-critical females are and how easily women feed into what others around them are doing. This doesn't exclude men from the influences of how others around them are eating, but the impulse is not as strong as it is for women.

What can we do to lessen the effect that the extremely processed and fried food choices of those around us have on our own choices? Focus on balance. Most of us have probably experienced resisting temptation and choosing a salad when our friend orders a burger. By the time the meal is over, we've eaten half of our friend's fries and are still craving a burger, which we then end up eating a few days later, anyway. If everyone around you is ordering a burger and you are in the mood for one (or just admittedly are influenced by those around you), order a burger.

This is the first step in the CUSP method: concentrating on what your body is in the mood for. Instead of choosing a regular burger, maybe choose a veggie or turkey burger. This is the second step of CUSP: understanding what food groups make up that food you're in the mood for. Maybe ask for a side salad instead of fries. Add some extra fruits or veggies on the burger like pineapple (don't knock it until you try it), avocado or onions.

There you have it, the third step of CUSP: supplementing the meal with the food groups it was lacking. And lastly, the final step, portioning, will occur once the food is right in front of you. Consider how large the burger is. If it's the same size as your face, the portion is definitely too large. Maybe only eat half and save the other half for later.

The best part about this strategy is that in the same way unhealthy habits are contagious, so are healthy ones! If your friends see that you've ordered a side salad instead of fries, they may also switch to the salad or agree on only one order of fries for the table to split, rather than one order per person.

If Samantha had followed this strategy, her meal would have been more balanced, she wouldn't have forced herself to exert some crazy self-control that she would later give in to anyway, she would have felt way less guilty, and she would have encouraged her friends to make a few healthier decisions as well. It's a win, win, win, win and Samantha gets to enjoy a yummy burger! Don't let the unhealthy choices of those around you manipulate your food choices; instead, take an active role in helping encourage healthier choices all around.

* * *

CHANGES YOU CAN MAKE IN YOUR LIFE TODAY:

- Do not be easily influenced by unhealthy choices of others around you
- No need to force yourself to exert willpower to avoid that unhealthy influence
    - INSTEAD, CUSP it and craft a meal that you are in the mood for, but keep it balanced and as always listen to your body for healthy portion sizes

- Remember that with every healthy and balanced choice you make, you have the power to influence those around you

CHAPTER 12

THE COMPARISON DEVIL

IN THIS CHAPTER YOU WILL LEARN:

- Why it's unnecessary to compare what you eat to what someone else eats
- How following the CUSP method will help satisfy your body with what it needs, and it doesn't matter if what your body needs is different from what your friends' bodies need
- Why pushing your nutritional views on someone else is silly because what works for one person may not work for another

* * *

Erin was so happy she was hitting it off well with her roommate and the girls on her floor. It was only the second week of her freshman year of college, and she already felt like she had found some new lifelong friends. The girls did everything together, so of course, this included eating. Recently, Erin had been feeling a little bit weird about the way the girls discussed everything they ate, all the time. Her friends from high school rarely mentioned what they ate, and if they were eating together, they didn't go into any further details other than what they were ordering. Erin's friends from college, however, constantly seemed to be looking for approval on what they were eating. For example, if one of the girls chose a salad, she would have to mention that she was eating healthy that day. On the contrary, if another friend chose pizza, she would have to mention that she had been eating really healthy all week, as if she was attempting to justify eating pizza.

Who says that pizza should only be "earned" if you've eaten healthy all week? Why do we feel the need to brag every time we choose a salad? This is what I call the comparison devil. As humans, we seem to find it necessary to compare ourselves to others in hopes of receiving their approval. We assume that those around us will judge us if we choose pizza and will be proud of us if we choose salad.

In reality, no one really cares that much about what anyone else is eating; most people's primary concern is only what they themselves are eating. Rule #1 is to never comment on what someone else is eating. If they chose salad, good for them. If they chose pizza, also good for them. Intuitive eating is about listening to your body for what it needs. (Concentrate on what your body is in the mood for—am I getting repetitive yet?! Good. I want this method to really stick in your brain.) No one knows what your body needs except you. Of course, it's important for nutritional purposes to aim for your meals to be balanced (understand, supplement), but it doesn't have to be a black and white choice of pizza or salad, as Erin's friends made it seem. And no matter what Erin chooses as long as she doesn't overeat (portion), she isn't going to cause any detrimental health issues.

Maybe, if Erin's friend who chose the pizza also supplemented her meal with a side salad, she would be full from the salad, eat less pizza and therefore, feel less guilty. The self-approval and lack of guilt that she would feel would make her less inclined to discuss her food choice with everyone at the table. The same goes for her friend who chose the salad. Maybe if this friend also wanted to have a small slice of pizza on the side, she would have felt more satisfied after her meal, and again, this positive internal feeling would reduce the likelihood of her seeking outside approval from friends.

Another similar issue arises when people push their nutritional views on others. Maybe one of your friends has decided to follow a trendy new diet. She personally thinks this is best for her health and sees great results from it. Why does everyone around her need to know that she is on this diet, and why does she insist that everyone around her also try it? The motivation is similar. This person is seeking approval. Is the weight she lost noticeable? Are the sacrifices she is making worth it? Obviously, she is looking to you for these answers, which signifies that she may not feel satisfied with some area of her diet. (The odds are that her dissatisfaction stems from nutritional deprival, as most diets could be renamed "deprive yourself for a few weeks and lose weight" for a more literal interpretation.)

The best thing to do when you are with someone like the fictitious trendy dieter or Erin's friends is simply to ignore the talk about what others are eating. Sometimes, nutrition is like politics. Lots of people love to talk about it, but most of those people don't really know what they're actually talking about.

There are some central ideas that people believe, like people should have the right to vote for their president and vegetables are good for you. But, from there, all kinds of personal truths emerge. Just as two voters debate which president is a better candidate, two health-conscious people debate whether gluten is good for you or bad for you. In both cases, it depends on who you ask. An individual with celiac disease will not respond the same as someone who can easily process gluten.

The moral of the story is to treat talking about what someone else is eating the same way you treat talking about politics; just don't do it.

* * *

CHANGES YOU CAN MAKE IN YOUR LIFE TODAY:

- Stop commenting on what someone else at the table is eating and focus on your own meal (unless you're asking how it tastes or something else irrelevant to nutrition)
- Always follow CUSP to figure out what your body needs and don't worry whether or not this is different from someone else
  - Concentrate on WHAT YOUR BODY NEEDS
    - Key: this can be different for everyone
    - No matter what it is that your body is in the mood for, keep it balanced, keep it portioned
  - Make an effort to supplement your meal with additional fruits and veggies as often as you can

CHAPTER 13

WHAT INSPIRES HEALTHY HABITS?

IN THIS CHAPTER YOU WILL LEARN:

- What inspires the millennial generation to eat healthy
- The problem with individuals who eat junk frequently and still remain stick thin
- The most common motivators of food choice in America and how these have changed over the past 10 years
- How we can encourage healthier eating patterns based on these motivators
- Why so many Americans are on a "diet" yet at the same time are overweight or obese
- General BMI guidelines

- How following the CUSP method eliminates your need to exert willpower
- What a realistic timeline for weight loss looks like

* * *

Morgan looked at herself in the mirror and wasn't happy with who she saw staring back at her. She had let her unhealthy habits get a little out of hand recently. Finals had just begun and pop tarts on the way to the library were the peak of her nutritional intake for the day. The gym never fit into her busy studying schedule, and when her stress was too much to handle she turned to friends and one too many alcoholic drinks.

She decided that she didn't want to feel this way any longer. Morgan wanted to look in the mirror and be proud of her reflection. So, she decided to completely transform her lifestyle to a much healthier one. She woke up every morning and went to the gym before studying. Morgan packed healthy, balanced meals in a lunch box for the library, and only consumed moderate amounts of alcohol when relaxing with friends.

A few small changes added up to big results. She lost four pounds during her two weeks of finals and truly felt like herself again. She finally felt proud of the person staring back at her. However, Morgan wasn't going to stop there. She knew she had an additional 10 pounds or so that her body didn't need and to help lose this additional weight, she would continue to keep up these healthy habits.

Morgan exemplifies the most common reason that people in the millennial generation eat healthy, to lose or maintain weight. This can be a great thing. Often, weight is a signal for how healthy a person is. But, it can also be a very scary thing. This is because there are many times when weight provides no signal for how unhealthy a person is. You know that friend who has the highest metabolism known to man. I mean he or she can eat burger after burger and dessert every day and never gain a pound. In fact, sometimes that friend complains about "wanting to gain weight" and it makes you really angry, obviously because you're jealous.

Let's pause for a moment before we let the green-eyed monster cloud our view. If that friend is only motivated to eat healthy when they are unhappy with their weight, they will never be motivated to eat healthy. Which means people like this probably eat junk all the time with little or no regard to its impact on their health, since it doesn't impact the way their bodies look. I actually feel bad for someone like this, because there was a time in my life when that was me. And you know what, yes, I was skinny. But, no, my body didn't feel healthy. I often lacked energy and felt sluggish.

The medical term for this is "Metabolically Obese Normal Weight" and it's defined by a person who is not considered obese based on their height and weight but experiences many of the same conditions obesity brings, like being predisposed to type 2 diabetes, and other concerning health factors. This "Metabolically Obese Normal Weight" person is often a young person whose unhealthy habits have yet to catch up to him or her. This is the danger with millennials.

If the most common motivator of healthy eating is weight loss or maintenance, what about everyone else? Liz Sanders, Associate Director of Food Communications for the International Food Information Council (IFIC) explained to me that, "Weight loss and eating to manage a chronic condition were two of the reasons why people made healthier choices. When you're young, you often won't be experiencing those chronic conditions that are going to immediately change the way you eat." Therefore, without that motivation, young people who aren't attempting to lose or maintain weight but who do eat healthy, often do so to proactively avoid long-term complications. Unfortunately, this is quite uncommon (basically, I'm one in a million).

It's extremely difficult for millennials to see a direct correlation between the food choices they make and their future risks of many cancers and diseases. At an age where you feel invincible, it seems almost impossible to try to imagine how what you choose for dinner may lessen the future risk of developing certain health conditions.

What can we do for millennials to help encourage healthier eating even when not attempting to lose or maintain weight? In general, American's food choices are motivated first by taste, then by price, then by healthfulness. Check out the graphic below from the IFIC's 2015 Food and Health Survey.

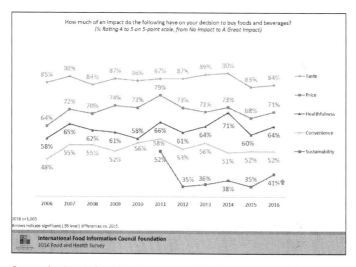

© International Food Information Council Foundation 2016. Re-used with permission.

With taste being the obvious top motivator, the more overlap there is between what tastes good and what is healthy, the more people will eat healthy. Have you ever been so impressed with how amazing a salad tasted? You could not even believe how good it was because you didn't know salad could taste that good. That is how I feel whenever I eat a Sweetgreen salad. I try to make this myself in my kitchen at home using similar ingredients, but I can never get it just right. We need more healthy eateries that taste good on college campuses and in areas densely populated with young professionals.

Because price falls right behind taste (although decreasing in importance from 2014 to 2015), these tasty and healthy foods cannot be priced too high. This turns off price sensitive people who want to eat healthy. Healthy foods, however, do cost significantly more for a company to produce so having low prices would mean having very low profit margins, and in the business world, this would likely lead to companies going out of business. It's a thin rope that we must walk along to find the right balance of taste, price and healthfulness, but by increasing the number of options that are available, we can only make a positive contribution to the health of Americans.

Also, note on the graphic the 9% decrease from 2014 to 2015 in the impact of healthfulness on food purchases. This is a quite concerning decrease. Another scary statistic from the survey is the sustainability category (the food waste issue is coming up yet again). From its peak in 2011 as an influencer of 52% of food purchases, it has decreased to 35% in 2015.

Social change to increase both of these numbers is necessary, and maybe if more people would eat the way I advocate for in this book, we can slowly make a difference. Just like the young man throwing starfish back into the ocean (if you've never read this story, pause and go read it now, it continuously inspires many aspects of my life), one person can make a difference. You are that person, and the time to transform your life is today. Not tomorrow or next week or on January 1st, but today.

What about Morgan? As a millennial who is concerned about her weight, she is already motivated to eat healthy. The more healthy options Morgan has around her, the easier it will be for her to continue to make smart choices. Morgan's stance on her body and weight loss goals are, in fact, the norm. Four out of five Americans are trying to lose weight or maintain their current weight. What! That's huge! That means that in a family of five, all but one are very carefully monitoring their weights. Why then, are 68.8% of American adults overweight or obese? How horrifying!

It's partly due to the fact that more than half of these overweight and obese Americans see themselves as being in excellent or very good health. If reading that last sentence made you a little nervous, you should probably take a few minutes to self-evaluate. Although not always an accurate picture of muscle mass, a quick online Body Mass Index (BMI) calculator can give you some idea of where you fall on the spectrum. The following guidelines are generally accepted. A BMI of 18.5-24.9 kg/m² is normal, 25-29.9 kg/m² is overweight, 30+ kg/m² is obese and 40+ kg/m² extremely obese. Just remember, BMI doesn't always tell you the whole story, so if you fall into a category you are confident must be wrong, try looking into your body fat percentage or waist circumference measurement and of course speaking with your doctor.

The other answer to the puzzle of why there is such a large number of individuals both watching their weight and at the same time remaining overweight or obese, is that people see a lack of their own willpower as being the number one reason why they cannot lose or maintain weight. Sure, there is some willpower involved in making healthy choices. When you think of what you want for lunch, do you choose a burger or a salad? That's a choice that you make with your own willpower.

But really, the problem is that willpower is a very small part of maintaining or losing weight. Because, like discussed throughout this book, if you want the burger, have the burger. (C of CUSP). Intuitive eating prevents future episodes of overeating. Rather than trying to assert your "willpower," craft a balanced meal (U and S of CUSP) based on the foods you are in the mood for and beware of portion sizes (P of CUSP).

Start with that burger. Would you mind switching from a

beef burger to a veggie, lentil, or turkey burger? (Hint: you don't have to say yes). If you would not enjoy a turkey burger, do not order one. You now have a protein, let's add a starch. Maybe put your burger on a whole wheat bun. Always try to choose complex carbohydrates when you can, like brown rice, whole wheat/grain bread or pasta. These are a better choice because of their high fiber content and slower digestion pace. However, if this swap will completely ruin the meal for you, it may not be worth it. (If you are not enjoying the healthy foods you are eating, you will quickly abandon your concern for the healthfulness of them. Food is meant to be enjoyed.)

Next, choose some veggies for your side. How about roasted asparagus? What a great way to supplement your meal. Don't forget the dairy, which is very easy in this case, just add cheese. Depending on how large this burger is, you may have to eat some now and save some for later. Now you have yourself a balanced meal that will satisfy your craving, and requires little "willpower." See how easy it is to CUSP it?

Most of the motivators of what we eat are subconscious, so try to get out of the mindset that you need to exert "willpower" to maintain a healthy diet. Instead, remind yourself to eat whatever you want, but always aim to consume balanced meals and keep in mind portions sizes. Remember all of the environmental factors that cause you to overeat, even when you don't want to, and tailor your environment to avoid getting caught in those traps. If you do this, I can pretty much guarantee you that you won't have any issues losing or maintaining weight. And yes, you can eat dessert.

As for Morgan, she will continue to be motivated by the way she looks. Although it's concerning that most of the ideal body images seen in the media are unrealistic, as long as Morgan continues to see her body growing stronger and shedding the unnecessary extra pounds, she will remain motivated to lose and eventually maintain her weight.

It's extremely important, however, that Morgan doesn't expect to lose weight too quickly. The number three reason (just behind willpower and lack of time) why people give up on their weight loss or maintenance journeys is not seeing results quickly enough. In the world we live in of instant gratification, especially for the millennial generation, the time it takes to lose weight in a healthy way is too slow for many Americans. One pound is about 3,500 calories. Divide this by seven days in a week, and you would need to have a caloric deficit of 500 calories per day compared to your pre-weight loss eating and exercise routine to lose one pound per week.

Because many people are not satisfied with only losing one pound in a week, undereating and then future overeating becomes a huge problem. Those expecting to be accelerating their weight loss mostly end up accelerating their weight gain.

Being aware of potential roadblocks like the many mentioned in this chapter will make your weight loss and/or maintenance journey much smoother and more enjoyable. So buckle up and enjoy the ride! Remember- life is about the journey, not the destination.

* * *

CHANGES YOU CAN MAKE IN YOUR LIFE TODAY:

- Make healthy choices not just to change the way your body looks, but to prevent future cancers and diseases
  - Encourage that "metabolically obese normal weight" family member or friend to do the same
- Do a quick google search for a BMI calculator and see where you fall on the spectrum
  - Consider how following the CUSP method can help improve this number if necessary
- Give-up on "willpower" and transform your lifestyle to a healthier one that will help you stand out from the majority of people who can't keep off the weight they've previously lost (Hint: CUSP it…)
- Remember that good things take time. Rome wasn't built in a day. Your fabulous body won't be either
  - Set realistic weight loss goals

PART 5

PORTION

Don't you just hate it when you think you've done everything right, but the outcome still isn't what you were hoping for?

Like when you study so hard for a test, but you earn an average grade anyway. Or, when you prepare for hours on end for that meeting with your boss but you still don't impress him or her. Or, when you are so confident after that job interview, but a few weeks later you end up with a rejection email in your inbox.

There are many times in life when we try our hardest and still seem to fail. This is the case with most people who always seem to be on a diet. If their diet actually worked, they would no longer be on one. Life is hard. Unfortunately, there are going to be plenty more failures in our futures. But, your health does not have to be one of them. Because I'm not going to let it be.

I'm not going to let you be one of those people who tries and tries to lose weight but consistently fails. Or, one of those people who thinks they're super healthy, but goes to the doctor and finds out quite the opposite is true. Or, one of those people who admits they would love to lose a few pounds, but doesn't think it's worth the effort. All of these people have one thing in common. They make it too complicated for themselves. They forget the key step of the CUSP method. They fail to portion.

Notice that throughout this book I have never once called it "portion control." What did step one teach us about the way the human brain reacts to telling yourself that you can't have something? That it will backfire and we shouldn't control what we can and cannot have. So, don't stress about having to exert willpower and limit the amount of food you eat. That is not what portioning is about. It's about serving yourself the healthy amounts of food your body needs - nothing more and nothing less.

CUSP is not a set of rules that you MUST follow. Instead, CUSP teaches you how to think and make decisions regarding the foods you eat. Therefore, it's not that you absolutely must portion everything you eat. If one night, you want to eat a whole pint of ice cream because when you concentrate on what your body is in the mood for, you are craving ice cream, then go for it. You will not be wrong. You will not be failing at CUSP. If you listen to your body, you will never fail at CUSP.

However, what I've learned is that when you listen to your body, you will make it about ¼ of the way through that pint, and your body will tell you something like, "Thanks for loving me enough to listen to what I was craving and allowing me to enjoy this ice cream. However, I am full now, and if you continue to feed me more ice cream, I will begin to feel sick and you will begin to feel guilty. Now is a good place to stop."

I think you agree that you don't enjoy feeling uncomfortably full. Your stomach aches and you feel like it's about to explode. You immediately regret eating those huge portions. And, what I've found, is when I eat those huge portions and feel guilty, I fall back into cycles of binge eating and depriving my body, which is a place I never want to go again. But there's nothing you can do because the damage is already done.

Step four—portioning, will simply eliminate that feeling. You have already agreed that you don't enjoy that overfull feeling, so why put your body through it? Instead, serve your body the amounts of food that it needs. I promise your body will thank you. Be confident that if you give your all, you will succeed. (Thank you for that, CUSP.)

CHAPTER 14

THE DARK SIDE OF SOCIAL MEDIA

———

IN THIS CHAPTER YOU WILL LEARN:

- How seeing photos of food on social media can stimulate your appetite
- How we can take control of this dangerous relationship with food cravings and social media
- The positive impact social media and other apps can have on our health

* * *

Dylan was sitting at the kitchen table of his college apartment scrolling through his Instagram feed, just after finishing dinner.

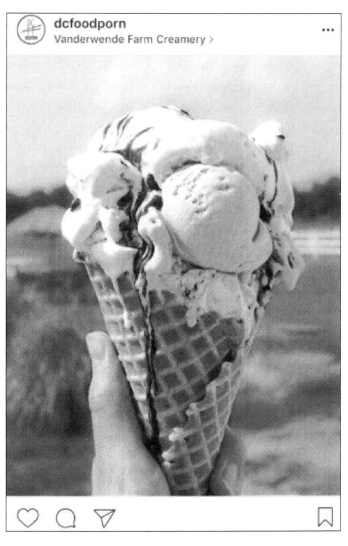

dcfoodporn
Vanderwende Farm Creamery >

⋯

♡ ◯ ◁ ◫

dcfoodporn
Bethesda Bagels >

•••

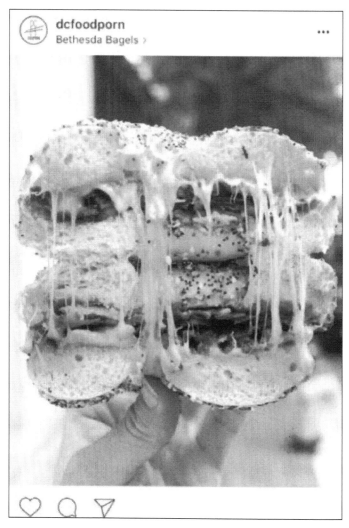

© Justin Schuble 2016. Re-used with permission.

His eyes landed on "dcfoodporn's" latest post. Words could never do this sweet photo justice, so I've reproduced it on the left below. I want you to feel the same feelings that Dylan felt when seeing this photo in his feed, so I've also chosen another image from the same account, in case you're more of a foodie than a dessert lover.

As he stared at the chocolate sauce melting and dripping down the sides of the oozy ice cream cone, Dylan's mouth began to water. "The things I would do to eat that ice cream cone right now," he thought to himself.

"Hey Jim," Dylan shouted across the kitchen to his roommate. "How about we go out for some ice cream tonight?" "Hmmmm," Jim thought to himself. "Yeah! I could go for some ice cream right about now. Let's do it."

And just like that, seeing just one post on social media motivated Dylan to convince his roommate within a matter of seconds to go out and get some ice cream. Professor Levitsky described to me the many ways in which people are exposed to food stimuli, which include anything from social media, vending machines, or TV commercials.

Dr. Gene-Jack Wang, Chairman of the Brookhaven National Laboratory Medical Department, and his colleagues studied how food stimuli affect the brain. They found, "The marked increase in brain metabolism by the presentation of food provides evidence of the high sensitivity of the human brain to food stimuli. This high sensitivity coupled with the ubiquitousness of food stimuli in the environment is likely to contribute to the epidemic of obesity."

This means that when we see photos of food on social media, we are much more likely to crave and later eat these foods. Have you ever been craving some random food for days and were wondering where that craving came from? You probably scrolled past a picture of it without even consciously realizing it.

I'm not here to bash social media food accounts. In fact, dcfoodporn is awesome. It's one of my favorite Instagram accounts. I love learning about new trendy eateries to check out. I also love Facebook recipe videos like the ones on Buzzfeed's "tasty" account. They help me add diversity to my often uninteresting college student meals.

However, it is crucial to understand the impact of the constant inundation of photos of food on our eating habits. So you follow some dessert food account on Instagram. Should you unfollow it? I would say absolutely not. Your friend, who knows you are a dessert lover, is regularly going to be tagging you in these photos anyway, and if you don't see them on that account, you're likely to see similar ones that your grandma shared on Facebook.

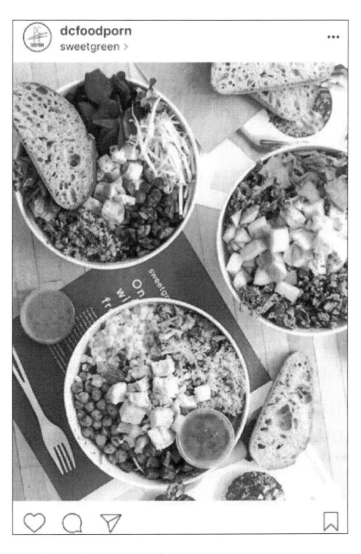

dcfoodporn
sweetgreen >

© Justin Schuble 2016. Re-used with permission.

We can't run from the world we live in. We can't be afraid of our own shadow. We can't label foods as "good" or "bad" and continuously avoid those we deem "bad." We need to accept the world as it is today and adapt our lifestyle to live in this world, in a healthy way. Should Dylan have exerted "willpower" after seeing the photo of the ice cream and decided not to go? Maybe, if he already had ice cream at lunch and knew that it would make him feel sick. But, if Dylan really wanted the ice cream, it's all about balance. (He was following the CUSP method—his body was in the mood for it). He should enjoy his treat and remember the importance of portioning. It's best for Dylan to order a small.

Dylan should keep in mind, that he was likely influenced by a social media post. If later that night, Dylan felt some sort of guilt for eating the ice cream, as he was watching his weight and knows dessert probably isn't helping, he should think back to why he wanted the ice cream in the first place. Scrolling through Instagram as soon as he finished dinner was probably not the best way to avoid seeing dessert stimuli.

Next time, if Dylan does want to avoid eating dessert after dinner, he can simply avoid social media for a half hour or so until his post-dinner dessert cravings dissipate. What? Thirty minutes of no social media! Yes, you can do it. I am not even mimicking millennials here, because I am one myself. Thirty minutes of no social media can be hard. But the fact that I even typed that sentence is a quite concerning example of our generation's dependency on technology.

There is, however, good news! Social media is not all bad. In fact, many of those same food accounts that post pictures of high calorie meals and desserts, also post very healthy and balanced meals. See the dcfoodporn Instagram below.

In addition to these healthy posts by popular food accounts, there are thousands of health and fitness accounts across all social media platforms. These make finding a new workout or recipe as easy as the click of a button. The digital world expands much further than just social media, with all kinds of workout and calorie tracking apps that you can tailor to your specific needs, preferences or goals. According to the IFIC, "36 % of Millennials are using an app or other means to track daily food and beverage intake, compared to 22 % of the population."

Just like we talked about accepting the bad and appreciating the good with Julie's Thanksgiving dinner, the same concept applies to social media. Sometimes, you just have to be aware that the picture of the bagel is going to linger in your mind and stir up some internal desire for a bagel that five minutes ago hadn't even crossed your mind. (Am I right on that one? Have you still been thinking about that bagel?)

Be aware of the dangers of social media and the impact photos have on your eating habits. Be conscious of your hunger levels (or desire for dessert like Dylan experienced) when scrolling through your Instagram feed. Promise yourself that you will take just as much good out of social media, if not more, than you do bad. That means download a fitness app, go for a run and track it, or look up how many calories are in an avocado before you eat the whole thing. You have thousands of resources at your fingertips. It's up to you how you choose to use them. I suggest you choose more of the good and less of the bad.

* * *

CHANGES YOU CAN MAKE IN YOUR LIFE TODAY:

- Follow more healthy food and lifestyle accounts on social media
  - Like @cusp_it on Instagram!
- Avoid social media at times of the day where cravings normally hit you
  - 3 p.m. during the workweek (if the midday slump and cravings hit you hard)
  - The first 30 mins after dinner (if you are a big dessert eater)
- When you do see a post for a sweet treat that you end up deciding to go out for, practice CUSP and be sure to be aware of the portion size
- Download and try out some new fitness apps
  - Go for a run or a walk and track it on a newly downloaded app

CHAPTER 15

STRESSED IS DESSERTS SPELLED BACKWARDS

———

IN THIS CHAPTER YOU WILL LEARN:

- Why your unhealthy cravings peak during times of high stress
- What the hormone cortisol is and why it's important
- How much an unhealthy diet decreases productivity
- How much a lack of exercise decreases productivity
- Ideas of ways to lower stress levels
- How the CUSP method applies to stress eating

＊ ＊ ＊

Ben cozied up in a local coffee shop with a latte, cinnamon raisin bagel and four papers to write. It was going to be a long day (and night) to say the least. A few hours had passed and although not sure if he was bored or hungry (but not really caring either way) he ordered himself "cup-of-noodles" and a chocolate chip muffin. One paper down. Soon enough, he was dying for another snack. Doritos and a Twix would have to do. The rest of his paper writing experience continued in a very similar manner. Every time Ben hit writers block, he immediately felt a craving for another snack or meal. He had to finish his papers, so he just had to give in to his cravings. Besides, midterms were only one week of each semester and he would be through them soon enough. Ben wasn't too concerned with the impact on his health of eating poorly for just one week.

The danger is that for the majority of college students, unhealthy habits continue to worsen as a given semester continues. Dr. Wansink studied this trend and found that when a semester began (for both fall and spring) students generally ate healthy. As the semester went on, he saw a steady decline in the amount of healthy foods purchased and a steady increase in the amount of unhealthy foods purchased. When the next semester began, the trend reset back towards healthy habits and then repeated itself.

College students know that busy schedules never really get better. The semester starts and there are no midterms, very few projects, and only occasional club meetings. As it continues, life begins to turn a lot more hectic. You have midterm after midterm after midterm, five group projects in one week, and three club meetings at the same time.

Stressed is an understatement. Junk foods require little preparation and when you're short on time; they're a great go-to. And, who wants a salad when you're feeling extremely anxious about the exam you have in the morning. Pizza, fries and a milkshake sounds way more comforting. After all, they are known as "comfort foods" for a reason.

If it makes you feel any better about all of the times you've stress eaten your feelings, just know that you really couldn't help yourself because stress biologically causes us to crave more fatty and sugary foods. It has something to do with the hormone cortisol. Stress alters this hormone's normal patterns of secretion. Nutritional Biochemist, Dr. Shawn M Talbott, puts these facts quite simply. He says, "The bottom line? More stress = more cortisol = higher appetite for junk food = more belly fat."

Unfortunately for Ben, due to his cortisol levels caused by the stress of his four papers, he probably was gaining more weight than he normally would have eating those same foods with no stress at all. Regardless of the weight gain aspect, let's look again at Ben's food choices. In a high stress situation, when you are pressed for time to meet deadlines, don't you want your body to function the best it can? Do you want to feel tired, sluggish, and irritable as you're trying to finish an important school assignment or task for work in a time crunch? Of course you don't.

No one wants to feel that way (ever) but especially at a time when you truly need all of your energy. Not even drinking four coffees could counteract the lack of energy Ben felt as a result of his poor food choices. We've all been in Ben's position at some point or another. We stress eat because we have deadlines to meet and we regret not making healthier choices when all we want to do is cuddle up for a nap instead of the work that needs to be finished ASAP. Why, then, after having this experience one time, do we avoid choosing better options to fuel our bodies in the future, at the times when we need it most?

We just can't help it! The increased levels of cortisol literally cause our bodies to long for those sugary and fatty foods we end up choosing. But, in the end, we do have a choice. We all want to be successful in school and in our careers. The food choices you make in high stress situations have a direct correlation with your performance. By enjoying balanced meals rich in fruits, vegetables, fiber and complex carbs, you will immediately feel higher energy levels, improved mood, and increased productivity.

A study, published by Population Health Management in 2012,

of just under 20,000 employees working for a variety of geographically dispersed companies, found that employees with an unhealthy diet were 66% more likely to experience a loss in productivity compared to those who ate healthy, balanced diets. Further, this same study found that employees who reported only exercising occasionally were 50% more likely to report lower levels of productivity than counterparts who reported regular exercise. Look better, feel better, and do better at work, what else do you really want? Make the right decisions in high stress situations and your mirror, your body and your boss will thank you.

Focus on ways you can lower your stress levels. The lower your stress levels become, the more normal your cortisol secretion will become. You'll begin to see fewer cravings for those junk foods and consequently see less weight gain. Exercise, talk about what is causing you stress with friends and family, write down your feelings, practice yoga or other forms of meditation, listen to music, and lastly, what I find to be the quickest form of stress relief is self-reflection.

My mom read a magazine article about stress management when I was about 15 years old that completely transformed my life. It said, "If it's not going to matter in five years, don't spend more than five minutes upset by it." Obviously this is easier said than done, but since that day, anytime I am overly stressed or upset about a situation, I picture my life five years from now. Nine times out of ten, I was likely sobbing over something that would have absolutely no impact on my life, even in one year.

Another way I like to self-reflect during stressful times is to be thankful. I think about all of the amazing people that I have been blessed with in my life, and I know that even if I have nothing else besides those people, I will live a happy life. Try using both of these self-reflection tactics, in addition to other personal ways to relieve stress, and you won't end up emotionally eating your anxiety like Ben did.

If, however, you do end up turning to food to relieve your stress, just remember that it is a form of emotional eating. In the same way that Kyle ate his feelings in celebration of his "A," Ben ate his feelings in anticipation of his large workload ahead. As discussed with Kyle, emotional eating can be okay because you are a human being and humans eat emotionally.

Congratulations! I'm so glad you're not one of those aliens or robots. I was concerned for a moment. But really, all you can do in a situation like Ben's, is be aware of your emotional influences (in this case- stress) and do your best to resolve the problem from its root, which should rarely be through food. Concentrate on your body and its desires. Don't be too hard on yourself during high stress situations. It's the opposite of what you need. If you do end up eating as a result of stress, understand what types of food you are eating and how you can supplement them with additional nutrients. Lastly and most importantly, portion that meal or treat. Do not overeat because of stress; you will end up regretting it.

Don't let stressful times be your excuse to put on ten pounds because you allowed a box of pizza to be your punching bag. You're better than that. Go to the gym and actually punch a real punching bag. You'll be happier, stronger, and more productive.

* * *

CHANGES YOU CAN MAKE IN YOUR LIFE TODAY:

- Learn how to manage stress in ways that do not revolve around eating
  - Exercise (do I even need to write it anymore at this point?)
  - Meditate
  - Talk it out with family and friends
  - Write down what is bothering you
  - Listen to music
- Ask yourself if whatever you are stressed about will matter in five years
  - If the answer is no, do your best to deal with the stress and then let it go
- Self-reflect on the many things you have in life to be thankful for

- Focus on exercise and a balanced diet to see incredible productivity increases at work
- When you do stress eat, follow the CUSP method and focus on portions

CHAPTER 16

THE DANGEROUS CYCLE

IN THIS CHAPTER YOU WILL LEARN:

- Why restrictive diets don't work
- How weight loss impacts your metabolism
- The real reason you're on a diet but still not losing weight
- The importance of exercise that builds muscle
- How to prevent binge eating

* * *

Maria was having trouble losing weight. Her eating habits seemed normal compared to friends, but nothing would make the scale budge. She would go days monitoring everything she ate and was sure she had consumed less than 1200 calories. If she could not lose weight eating a low-calorie diet, she figured that she could never lose weight.

Generally, she restricted what she ate Monday through Friday. She almost always stuck to less than 1200 calories per day. Except for some Fridays, because on Friday nights she went out to a local bar near campus with her friends. She usually had a few beers there, but Maria would attempt to save space in her 1200 calories for the beer she was going to drink as well. So, if she was planning on drinking three light beers, she would only eat 900 calories that day. Saturdays and Sundays were her "cheat days" where she would go all out with the assumption that calories don't count.

Sadly, Maria's eating habits are extremely concerning. The first issue to address is her restriction of calories. When eating a low calorie diet, your metabolic rate will slow down. This slowdown is often less than people think, but it does occur. People who lose a large amount of weight usually feel the effects of metabolic slow down the most.

Depending on your age, weight, height and activity level, your body needs a specific number of calories to maintain its current weight. Eating fewer calories than this level will often result in quick weight loss. However, once you reach a lower weight, the number of calories your body needs to maintain this new weight will be lower than it previously was. Therefore, to continue losing weight, you will need to continue to cut calories. If Maria already lost a significant amount of weight, this could be influencing her current weight loss plateau.

Another problem for Maria could be that she is potentially underestimating the amount of calories she actually consumes in one day. As we know, estimating serving sizes is quite the challenge, so if her caloric measurements are based on eyeball estimates, she could be estimating a couple hundred less calories than she is actually consuming.

Or, Maria's problem could be in her exercise routine. Maybe she is only doing cardio and not focusing on any muscle building workouts. For the women reading this, I promise you won't "bulk up" if you decide to lift weights, or do body weight exercises. Unfortunately, female bodies cannot build muscle as quickly and as easily as male bodies can. Muscle cells need more energy than fat cells, so they burn more calories, even when you're not exercising. Building muscle can both increase your metabolism and benefit your heart and bones.

Another issue to consider in Maria's diet is her alcohol intake. Alcohol consumption in itself is always something to consider in terms of your health. It's not inherently bad, of course. Some studies even point to health benefits of moderate alcohol consumption, like the reduced risk of heart disease, ischemic stroke, and diabetes. However, the thing to keep in mind here is that this is moderate consumption, which means up to one drink per day for adult women of all ages and for men over age 65 and up to two drinks per day for adult men under age 65. Of course, this is not the typical drinking pattern of a college student, a young professional, or even for parents and grandparents.

Alcohol consumption usually does not occur in moderation. Instead, there are periods of no consumption, often during the week, and periods of high consumption, often on weekends. This isn't me telling you not to have your fair share of beers on a Friday night if you would like, but keep in mind the health consequences. It might not be necessary to drink on Saturday if you already had enough to drink on Friday.

You can think of alcohol the same way you think of dessert, following the CUSP method. You may not be supplementing your drink with high amounts of nutrients, but you have to make sure you portion it. Alcohol can be your angel and your devil; you just have to find the right balance.

It is critical that students do not reduce their caloric consumption significantly when they plan on drinking. First, this is going to cause the alcohol to take effect faster since there is less food in your stomach to help absorb it. And, because you will likely feel drunk even from a small amount of alcohol, your willpower will be nonexistent. Soon enough, you will end up with a slice of pizza the size of your face. So much for that 1200-calorie diet.

In addition to these potential hindrances to Maria's weight

loss, it is pretty obvious where the root of Maria's problems lies. In fact, many people who claim to be struggling with losing weight even on a low calorie diet face this same problem. It's a lack of satisfaction followed by a development of cravings, and lastly binge eating many more calories than were originally allowed by the restrictive low calorie plan.

This is exemplified by Maria's weekend "cheat days." Say Maria was truly sticking to 1200 calories per day for five days per week. Then, on the weekends where she really overdid it, she consumed 3000 calories each day for two days. Her total caloric intake for the week would be 12,000 calories, but she would be consuming the same amount of calories she consumed in all five weekdays combined, in just two weekend days.

Think of it like this, would you rather eat seven cookies on a Sunday evening or eat one cookie after dinner every single night of the week? Maria's calories work that same way. But, eating one cookie every day would be much easier for Maria's body to process. She could be eating over 1700 calories per day, every day for the same weekly caloric intake as before. If she maintained this caloric intake, Maria would rarely have cravings that went above her caloric allotment, and if they did, they sure wouldn't be more than double her daily intake as they were before.

By following the CUSP method and allowing yourself to eat

that cookie you may be in the mood for, you will not experience episodes of binge eating. In fact, by focusing on portions, overindulgence will rarely if ever occur.

The purpose of Maria's story is to better understand that a calorie restrictive diet leads to overeating. That being said, I'm not a fan of counting calories in general. It's good to have an awareness of how many calories your body burns in a day and how many you generally consume, but obsessing over every single calorie is a slippery slope that can lead to eating disorders, and therefore one that I will not promote.

The cycle Maria put her body through is extremely exhausting. One that if you have ever been in, I'm sure you can vouch for. Why only allow yourself to have dessert on the weekend, when you may just be in the mood for it on a Wednesday and not Saturday? Eating mindfully means to listen to your body's cravings when they naturally occur, not based on some schedule. Stop trying to exert that "willpower" and listen to your body. You will be surprised how amazing it feels when you do.

∗ ∗ ∗

CHANGES YOU CAN MAKE IN YOUR LIFE TODAY:

- Stop obsessing over counting calories
- Stop telling yourself what foods you can and can't have

- ◆ Instead, concentrate on what your body is in the mood for
- Do not plan "cheat days"—allow yourself those "bad" foods any day, any time
  - ◆ Serve yourself one portion and listen to your body for cues of satisfaction afterwards
- If you are attempting to lose weight but have been experiencing a plateau, consider possible reasons for this:
  - ◆ A slowdown of your metabolic rate due to recent weight loss
  - ◆ Your exercise routine
    - Supplement your cardio with muscle building exercises as well
  - ◆ The thousands of calories you drink in alcohol
    - Allow yourself to enjoy alcohol when in the mood but aim to portion your alcohol intake the same way you portion your food intake
  - ◆ The disastrous impact of those "cheat days"
  - ◆ The intense cravings that develop after depriving yourself and the additional binges that result

CHAPTER 17

BREAKING NEWS: DIETS DON'T WORK

———

IN THIS CHAPTER YOU WILL LEARN:

- More about why restrictive diets don't work for long-term weight management for many people
- Why so many people who lose weight end up gaining it all back plus more
- The problem with classifying foods as "good" or "bad"
- Why CUSP is a better option than dieting (if you don't already know)
- The importance of carbohydrates in our diets
- Why you shouldn't go gluten-free if you don't have celiac disease or a gluten intolerance
- The many benefits we gain from eating fats

- The role of sugar in our diets
- What happens to your body when you cut out a food group

* * *

Emma desperately wanted to lose weight. She was halfway through her freshman year of college and was not happy with the stereotypical freshman 15 that she had gained. She knew friends in the past who went on diets that involved cutting out almost all carbs, sugars, and fats. Basically, they ate only lean meats, veggies and some fruit.

Emma did a quick internet search and read about people who followed similar diets and lost weight quickly. This was exactly what she was looking for. A quick fix that she could focus on while she was home on winter break, so that by the time she was back at school she would already have reached her ideal weight.

What actually happened for Emma was, however, quite different. The initial pounds dropped quickly. She had lost about 10 pounds in two weeks sticking to a very strict low carb, sugar and fat diet. She was so proud of herself for having enough willpower to stick to the diet. No sweets, no burgers, no pizza. It did get old, but she was only planning to keep it up until she arrived back at school.

The first day Emma was back from break loving her transformation, she went a little overboard on the junk and sweets. Chocolate chip pancakes for breakfast, a Hershey's bar at 11 a.m., pizza for lunch, mac and cheese for dinner and a brownie with ice cream for dessert. But hey, she was 10 pounds thinner. She could afford to have a little treat, right? Emma dreamed about all of the foods she suppressed cravings for while she was dieting. She simply could not help herself from indulging in every pasta, cookie, and french fry that was in front of her. This binge eating, however, lasted a lot longer than her two-week diet did.

Four weeks had gone by and Emma had not only gained back the 10 pounds that she had lost, but she also gained an additional five pounds. She felt absolutely hideous. How could she have let this happen? Emma felt that she HAD to go on another diet. So, she did just that. It was back to unsatisfying meals of something like chicken and broccoli twice a day every day. Emma had fallen into a dangerous cycle of dieting, quite similar to the one Maria was stuck in.

Emma is an example of a person who found little success in a diet in terms of long-term weight loss or maintenance. If you tell yourself, "I have a party, wedding, formal etc. that I need to lose five pounds for, and afterwards I know I will gain those five pounds back and I'm okay with that," then sure, go on a diet. There's nothing wrong with that. But, for your health or even just your confidence, if you're trying to maintain a certain weight, diets will often not help you do that. In a study performed by Dr. Wansink, only 8% of people reported their most recent diet to have lasted longer than three months.

The first problem with diets is that they label foods as either "good" or "bad." Robyn Filpse, RD explained to me her belief that, "There really is a problem if you think some foods are healthy and some foods are bad because too much of anything is too many calories." Although calories are not the only thing that matters in terms of your overall health, they do play a very important role. That means that yes, it is possible to eat too many vegetables.

If you ate six plates of broccoli for dinner, it would be about the same amount of calories as if you were to eat two bowls of ice cream. Of course, broccoli has many more nutrients and health benefits than ice cream does, so in this situation, I would recommend choosing the broccoli, but in terms of weight loss or maintenance, you wouldn't notice a huge difference in this swap.

Intuitive eating does not focus on the good or bad in foods, but instead it focuses on what your body is in the mood for (by now I hope you recognize that this is the C of the CUSP method). Your goal should be to identify the macronutrients that are inside your food choice (this is the U), and incorporate additional nutrients and fibers where you can to make your meal balanced (this is the S). Lastly, to prevent overeating, make sure you serve healthy portion sizes (this is the P).

By allowing yourself to have the foods you are in the mood for, unlike Emma, you can fuel weight loss or maintenance without the long term weight gain that almost always results from strict diets.

Dr. Jim Painter explained to me that the idea of a diet is really a flawed concept. Many "diet" foods like low fat alternatives replace fat with sugar and other unhealthy ingredients, plus they make you feel less satisfied and more likely to overeat as a result. Take, for example, diet sodas. These artificially sweetened drinks trigger insulin, sending your body into fat storage mode.

Unlike non-diet soda, which would relieve your body's craving for sweets, diet sodas tend to leave you feeling less satisfied and more likely to reach for another soda or other junk foods to get that sugar fix your body wants. The worst part is diet sodas also dehydrate you, leaving you more irritable and tired. You should think twice next time you choose the low calorie or low fat food without taking a closer look at the ingredients.

Now, let's take a deeper look at Emma's diet and the food groups she has chosen. She claims she is eating lots of vegetables and that she is on a low carb diet. However, Emma doesn't know that carrots, onions, peas, and corn are all vegetables that are pretty starchy, especially the last two. Emma has eaten a lot of these veggies recently. And, that's not a problem. These veggies are filled with many essential nutrients. But, to really understand a balanced diet, it's key to understand which vegetables have the largest content of carbohydrates.

While we're on the carbohydrates issue, we see Emma cutting out essential nutrients that come from complex carbohydrates like whole wheat bread, whole wheat pasta, brown rice, quinoa, sweet potatoes, etc. These foods are indispensable to Emma's health, and she completely ignores them. Of course, Emma's body craves the levels of carbohydrates that it needs to function, and then she turns to simple carbs like white bread, pasta, and rice, to satisfy this.

Oh and if you don't have a gluten intolerance or celiac disease, going gluten free isn't going to help you lose weight. It might help you eat less carbs (although you could just overindulge in rice and gluten free breads and pastas), but that would lead to the same problem Emma is having with cravings. It would have been a much better choice for Emma to include more carbs in her diet and reduce the very high risk of future overeating.

What about fats? Emma said she doesn't eat many fats. Just this week, however, Emma enjoyed an avocado for breakfast one morning and salmon for dinner another evening. These, in fact, are fats! Yes... these "superfoods" are filled with fat!!! How is that possible? It's true that fats are higher in calories per gram than carbs or protein, but the logic that restricting your body from these foods will result in lower calories automatically, and thus, a healthier diet is misguided.

First of all, fats are absolutely essential in our diets. They help our bodies with digestion, managing inflammation, storing energy, ensuring proper functioning of our nerves and brain and regulating many bodily processes, among other things. When our body digests carbohydrates (from sugar or starch), our body breaks this down into glucose. Glucose may be stored in the form of glycogen or in adipose tissue-what you know as fat. This is the fat you think of when you look down at your stomach and see those extra rolls you are trying to lose (not to be too graphic).

This is not the same as the fat that is removed when you buy skim milk. Many people think that when they drink whole milk (which has fat in it), the fat immediately stores as fat inside their bodies. But in reality, quite the opposite is true. In Time Magazine, Alice Park explains, "Since full-fat dairy products contain more calories, many experts assumed avoiding it would lower diabetes risk. But studies have found that when people reduce how much fat they eat, they tend to replace it with sugar or carbohydrates, both of which can have worse effects on insulin and diabetes risk." In fact, fat can help slow down the insulin spike from sugar. So, you are better off eating a full fat dessert over a fat-free one.

Of course, not all fats are created equal. Many people by now have heard about the health benefits of fatty foods like the ones Emma included in her diet. These are commonly referred to as omega-3 fatty acids. Some of the many health benefits of these fats include but are not limited to: improved eye health, help fighting depression and anxiety, promotion of brain health during pregnancy, lower risk of heart disease, reduced ADHD symptoms in children, reduced symptoms of metabolic syndrome, help fighting autoimmune diseases, help fighting inflammation, improved mental disorders, help fighting Alzheimer's Disease, reduced fat in the liver, improved bone and joint health, and may help in preventing cancers.

Even if you just let your eyes skim over that very long list, you get the point that these fats can do amazing things for our bodies and our health. Still, even with the great reputation these fats have, people are pretty misinformed about them. The IFIC reports, "64 percent of Millennials rate omega-3 fatty acids, a type of polyunsaturated fat, as healthful, yet only 17 percent of Millennials rate polyunsaturated fats as healthful." But, we are getting there. Slow and steady wins the race. Don't be misinformed like Emma. Know what types of food you are putting into your body. This will help you make informed decisions about nutrition, so you are able to create a balanced meal.

Fats and carbs were not the only macronutrients Emma claimed to be cutting from her diet. The last was added sugars. We do know that added sugars are not the most healthful choice as they spike our insulin levels. We also know that fruit is very healthy for us to consume. In her diet, Emma was eating plenty of apples, bananas, and strawberries. These fruits do have sugar in them, but the sugar is a natural source of fructose bundled with fiber, water, vitamins, minerals, and antioxidants. As long as you're not overeating a ridiculous amount of fruit, I would not worry too much about natural sugar from fruits and vegetables, as those are not added sugars.

What Emma is right about, is that added sugars can be detrimental to our health. The American Heart Association's recommendation for the amount of added sugar a person should consume per day is no more than six teaspoons for women and nine for men. However, the average American consumes 22 teaspoons of added sugar per day. I don't know about you but picturing all that excess sugar is a bit sickening to me.

Keep in mind though, that Emma's diet of "low sugar" did not work out for her. Just like with all of the other food groups she attempted to cut out of her diet, Emma experienced intense cravings and ended up binge eating. If she would have allowed herself that one slice of cake when she may have wanted it (concentrate), she would not have felt the urge to eat four slices a week later (lack of portioning). It's all about balance (understand and supplement). You must really be catching on now!

Emma caused herself more weight gain than weight loss. Raise your hand if you've done the same at some point in your life. (Literally raise it. Admit it. I don't care if you're in a coffee shop or on the beach or somewhere else in public and people will look at you funny. Acknowledge to yourself that diets don't work because you have been in Emma's shoes before.) I know I have.

Nutritionist Allison Tepper worked in Georgetown University's dining hall (yes she was my incredible nutritionist; you have a stellar memory). She saw hundreds of students just like Emma. Allison taught me the idea that, "If you cut out a food group, your body can't function normally. If you cut out carbohydrates, your body starts to break down protein and then your metabolism slows down. So that's why people gain weight after a restrictive diet. You thought you were doing something good, but it backfired." So stop trying trendy diets. Stop trying to cut out food groups. Stop looking for a quick fix. Your body deserves better than that.

* * *

CHANGES YOU CAN MAKE IN YOUR LIFE TODAY:

- Never go on a diet again
  - Unless you are trying to lose weight for a specific occasion and are okay with gaining back the weight you lost
    - In that case, be my guest
- Stop labeling foods as unhealthy or healthy; it's not so black and white
- Instead of a diet, if you want to lose weight or lead a healthier life:
  - Listen to your body's cravings
  - Create a balanced meal out of those cravings
  - Always, always, always, be aware of portion sizes
    - This is the CUSP method reworded; I'm assuming you've really got it by now though
- Stop telling your friends that you're "cutting carbs" when you actually are eating plenty of carbohydrate-rich fruits and veggies
- And, stop trying to "cut carbs" because your body needs them
  - Instead, eat smart carbs—complex carbs like:
    - 100% whole wheat or whole grain bread and pasta
    - Sweet potatoes
    - Brown or wild rice
    - Beans (also great source of protein)
    - Oatmeal
    - Quinoa
    - Etc…

- ► I cannot write out all the complex carbs because there are so many out there; you have so many options and ways to spice up your starch in a healthy way—so take advantage
- Do not cut gluten in an attempt to lower your carb consumption
  - ◆ Cut gluten only when it's medically necessary
- Get over your fear of fat
  - ◆ Switch to whole milk or at least 2%
  - ◆ Stop eating fat-free desserts
  - ◆ And stop wasting money on fat free foods in general
    - ▪ Full fat = satisfied belly = easier to manage portions
- Be a little more aware of the amount of added sugars you consume daily and how much higher this is than the recommended six teaspoons for women and nine teaspoons for men
  - ◆ This doesn't include fruits—continue to enjoy the sweet sugars of nature

CHAPTER 18

USDA'S GENIUS GUIDELINES

———

IN THIS CHAPTER YOU WILL LEARN:

- About the MyPlate guidelines: The USDA's nutritional recommendations
- What your portions should actually look like
- How to apply MyPlate and the CUSP method to any meal
- Importance of snacking
- Why you should allow yourself to eat dessert

* * *

It's time to meet Rob. Rob is one of the lucky ones. Unlike many of the individuals we have discussed thus far, Rob doesn't need any of my advice. Rob already follows it all. He is the example of eating a healthy, balanced diet, and more than this, how he applies the same balance to all areas of his happy life. Rob simply CUSPs it!

Rob told me that his goal with everything he eats is to #1) enjoy foods he loves, #2) make sure he includes a variety of types of foods that his body needs (veggies, fruits, protein, starch, fats, dairy) and #3) make sure he doesn't overeat past the point of being full. Rob eats dessert when he is in the mood for it, but rarely eats more than he needs to feel satisfied. Rob doesn't limit himself to eating only foods considered healthy, but instead freely allows himself to eat whatever he is in the mood for, as long as he incorporates it into a balanced meal and is sure not to serve himself overly sized portions.

Rob eats as soon as he feels physically hungry; this means he usually eats about two or three snacks per day in addition to his three meals. He doesn't religiously follow a guideline for how many meals or snacks he should eat, but instead Rob follows his hunger cues. One day Rob might eat five smaller meals and another day he may eat three normal sized (but remember normal sized is almost always not the size that you are served at a restaurant). Rob maintains a healthy weight through both his eating habits and his exercise routine.

Rob's balanced meals are based on the guidelines of the United States Department of Agriculture (USDA). This is known as the MyPlate method. The USDA explains, "MyPlate is a reminder to find your healthy eating style and build it throughout your lifetime. Everything you eat and drink matters. The right mix can help you be healthier now and in the future." So how does MyPlate do this? With the well-known graphic below! You may have seen this before as it continues to grow in popularity.

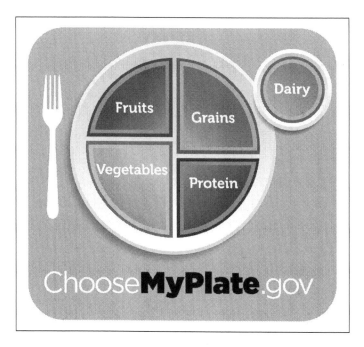

Credit: USDA 2011—Public Domain

As you can see above, MyPlate guidelines focus on five main food groups: fruits, vegetables, grains, protein, and dairy. The graphic shows the estimated amounts of each your plate should be filled with, every time you eat a meal. I like to think of it in the simplest way possible, that way applying it to my meals is as easy as 2+2 and I use the methodology no matter where I am.

I do that by aiming to fill about half of my plate with fruits and vegetables, ¼ with some sort of protein, and ¼ with some sort of grain or starch. On top of that, I aim to have some dairy and some fats within the meal as well. MyPlate is awesome because anything you are in the mood for can fit into this method.

All you have to do is CUSP it!

An example of a meal I am in the mood for as I type this is mac n cheese with broccoli (concentrate). What? You can eat mac n cheese as a healthy meal? Yes! You can! This is how I would craft this yummy balanced meal. I would cook 100% whole-wheat elbow noodles. This would be my starch (understand). I would make sure that I measured about ¼ of my plate or about one serving of pasta to cook (portion). That way, since I would be cooking exactly the right amount, I would not have to worry about portioning later.

Next comes the cheese. This is a food that gets a bad rep that it really does not deserve. Yes, many cheeses are high in calories and fat, but we know that #1) calories are not the only thing that matter #2) if you watch your portions, calories won't be an issue and #3) we need fat. Dairy is essential in our diets. Why do you think the USDA encourages us to eat dairy with every single meal! Side note—if you're lactose intolerant aim to get some of those essential nutrients like calcium, vitamin D, and potassium elsewhere.

Just like with the pasta choice, there are always choices you can make that are better for your health. So, for my cheese choice, I'd go with a type that is very high in protein, as this is going to be the protein of the meal. I would choose parmesan cheese that I will grate myself. Not only does grating cheese yourself taste better, but it also avoids extra additives that help de-clump the pre-shredded type. I would measure this grated cheese and add ½ cup into my pot. This would fill the ¼ protein requirement, the dairy requirement, and include the fat that I like to add into my meals as well (supplement and portion). Let's check out the nutrition info for the ½ cup of grated parmesan cheese, 19.2 grams of protein! I bet you're surprised. This is the equivalent of eating about two and a half eggs! All this protein for just 216 calories. This cheese really should be a competitor for some of the top protein bars on the market. The nutrition info is shockingly similar. It also has very low sugar. What more can you ask for?

Lastly, we need to fill the veggie part of our meal (supplement). I love the way broccoli tastes doused in melted parmesan cheese, so I would choose broccoli for my veggie. I would rinse one cup of broccoli, which would be a healthy serving that would fill about half of my plate (portion).

I would first steam the broccoli separately. I would then place it in the pot with the mac n cheese at the point when the pasta was close to being fully cooked. This gives just enough time to let the whole meal cook together and the cheese to seep into the broccoli, just the way I like it best. Once the whole meal is cooked, I will enjoy some lovely mac n cheese and I especially enjoy it more knowing that I had cooked a balanced meal.

See how easy (and tasty) the CUSP method is? You can enjoy any food in the whole world that you're in the mood for. You can easily recognize which food group it falls into and which it is lacking to help create a balanced meal. And lastly, by following the MyPlate guidelines, you now know what healthy portion sizes look like. It's easy as pie. And, you can still eat pie!

Something to note here is if you're looking for an excuse to act like you're "eating healthy" but carelessly overindulge, the MyPlate method isn't going to stop you. Technically, you could fill your plate with three large pieces of chicken in the protein section by stacking them, and still think you're following the guidelines. The point of MyPlate is to make eating healthy, balanced meals simple. So, there is not an extensive list of guidelines on how high each food should be stacked on your plate.

For those of you who are curious, one serving of chicken or meat should be about three ounces in size. This is about equivalent to a deck of cards. So, picture how tall a deck of cards is, that's about how tall the meat on your plate should be. Use that picture in your mind for your other food groups as well, and you will never have to worry about over-stacking.

If you are really following the CUSP method, portioning is crucial aspect. You cannot pull a fast one and over stack on CUSP, because we both know your body doesn't need that huge portion. If you are concentrating on what your body needs, you will learn to serve yourself healthy portions. Your body will feel the most nourished and energized when you do so. Therefore, by following the first step of CUSP, the last step will come naturally. It a learning experience, which is why we provide you with the MyPlate guidelines to make it as simple as possible for you.

At this point we have gone through balanced meals and how to construct them, but in the back of your mind the whole time you've been reading this chapter, you've been curious about Rob's habit of snacking. (People have always told me I should have become a mind reader. Unfortunately, it's not a college major.) The dieter inside of you is yelling, "Snacking is bad! Never snack!"

Please forget everything negative you ever thought about

snacking. You may be thinking to yourself, "Snacking means additional calories, and additional calories mean additional weight gain right?" Sure, if you think of nutrition as only calories in and calories out. (But we know it's more than that). However, just to silence that voice in your head, I will prove to you that incorporating snacks between meals will lead to a consumption of FEWER calories. That's right. Fewer! How so? It goes back to a similar idea of the deprivation diet. If you don't allow yourself to snack between meals, you will become ravenous before your next meal (unless your previous meal had enough calories for the whole day, and in that case you have other problems to tackle).

So, when it's finally time for that meal and you feel ravenous, you will eat as if you are competing in a race with everyone at the table to see who can finish their plates first for a 10 million dollar prize. (When I want to, I can eat realllllllyyyy fast with absolutely no regard to manners whatsoever. So, if I'm sitting at the table with you, you might as well just give up now.)

Obviously, when you eat at a very quick speed, you will overeat. You still feel hungry even after you finish your plate because it's been about four minutes and it will take your brain another 16 minutes to send the signal that you're full. So, you eat more. Because you were SO hungry, nutrition doesn't even count for this meal. You literally felt like you could have been starving to death. (But I promise you weren't. It does feel like that sometimes though, I have been there. One time I wolfed down a whole quesadilla in less than twenty five seconds. I told you I can eat fast.) These additional calories are much greater than the calories you would have consumed if you had just chosen to eat a small snack between meals.

In addition, the benefits span a much wider range than just caloric consumption. Snacking also can help avoid low blood sugar. Your blood sugar is glucose that flows through your bloodstream to be used as energy for your cells or stored for future use. As you may know, blood sugar levels are especially important for individuals with diabetes. When you have too much glucose, your blood sugar levels will be high and your body will store fat. When your blood sugar levels are too low, you may feel tired, shaky, hungry or irritable.

You have probably heard the advice to always eat breakfast. Blood sugar drops during the evening and early morning hours, while you are sleeping and not eating. When you wake up in the morning, your blood sugar is low due to an overnight fast. Eat breakfast and have snacks like Rob does. You will eat less at meals, have more energy, and feel less hungry throughout the day.

One more thing though, choose your snack carefully. For optimal nutritious benefits, aim for a snack of 200 calories or less (but don't obsess over calorie counting). Try to choose a snack that is not too high in sugar—always less than 10 grams and even that is a bit high. If you remember, total consumption of added sugar per day in women should only be about six teaspoons and nine in men. Also, chose a snack that is a combination of protein, carbohydrates, and fats. Aim to incorporate whole grain carbs as often as you can.

Try different snacks and see what works for you. I could give you a list of snacks that I love (like 1 tablespoon of peanut butter on an apple or a banana, 100% whole-wheat toast with ½ avocado spread across and topped with basil, or a few slices of white cheddar cheese on Triscuits) but everyone is different. We may have different taste buds or maybe you're two times my size and these snacks don't seem to fill you up. That's why you should not focus too much on counting the calories. As long as you rely on your body's hunger cues to help you portion, you don't have to worry about counting calories anyway.

As with everything we have been discussing, of course the CUSP method applies when choosing a snack. Always treat your body to what it is in the mood for. Think about how to craft a balanced snack and keep your portion in check. You will thank me later when you eat half as much as you used to at dinner, feel higher levels of energy throughout the day, and see those extra pounds disappearing.

One last lesson we can all learn from Rob is his view on dessert.

As we know, human willpower is not the way to live a balanced life. So, when craving dessert, Rob goes for it. Rather than holding himself back and continuing to think about it until he eventually overeats it, he goes for it as soon as he wants it. By doing this, Rob actually keeps the amount of dessert he eats relatively low, even though that seems counterintuitive. Satisfying cravings means you don't feel the need to eat four cookies at a friend's birthday party because you ate a cookie yesterday and aren't in the mood today. Follow the CUSP method for dessert, again listening to your body, making the dessert choice as balanced as you can and most importantly watching that portion.

However, as much as we all love dessert, calories can add up quickly. The best thing I ever did to help tame my very large sweet tooth was purchase individually wrapped small candies of my favorites kinds (like Hershey Kisses, Reese's, Rollo's and Werther's Original, but you can chose any mini-candies that you love). Whenever I finish a meal and want something sweet, I grab a single one of these candies, for example one Hershey's Kiss. I focus on truly enjoying the creamy flavors inside. Clinical Psychologist Dr. Jean Kristeller explains, "Our taste buds are chemical sensors that tire quickly. The first few bites of a food taste better than the next few bites, and after a large amount, we may have very little taste experience left at all." Savor those first few bites (in the case of a Hershey's Kiss, I make sure to take at least three small bites rather than one large).

Knowing that I can have another kiss after my next meal, deters me from having a strong desire to eat another. I enjoyed the yummy chocolatey taste, and I knew I could have another later if I was in the mood. The best part about this is obviously the portion size. One Hershey's Kiss is only 22 calories and less than three grams of sugar. If you're feeling especially healthy, choose the dark chocolate kiss or another dark chocolate candy, as these antioxidants can actually provide significant health benefits.

The other thing I do every time I want dessert is carefully scan my options. Then I ask myself, "Is that cookie worth it?" What I mean is, for those 200 calories, do I really want that cookie? If the answer is yes, I will absolutely go for it. But, if that cookie is not my favorite kind and I know it will just taste so-so, I personally don't want to "waste the calories." Think of it like this, the calories I eat are precious. If I'm going to eat dessert, it better be something really good. It better be my favorite kind of cookie, the kind that I continue to think back on how good it was for days. It's not that my calories are necessarily limited because I do not withhold myself from anything, but by eating balanced and portioned meals, I am not consuming thousands of excess calories per day. If I was, I would be overweight and I sure wouldn't be writing this book.

This concept comes back to satisfaction and experience. I used to eat any dessert that was in front of me. But, if it was something I didn't like that much, I wouldn't feel satisfied and I would continue to eat more dessert later that night or the next morning to find that satisfaction. Whereas now, I choose small portions of sweets I love, and I am easily satisfied by a small amount. By concentrating on what I really want, I get more satisfaction out of a smaller portion. Thank you, CUSP!

By eating mindfully and not adapting a diet mentality, you, just like Rob, can enjoy all your favorite foods and desserts whenever you like. The best part is that you will be in an optimal state of health, and applying this balance to other areas of your life (work-life balance, financial balance- what to save and what to spend, free time balance- when to go out and have fun and when to rest etc.) will help you live a happier life. Doesn't this sound like a scam or gimmick? Believe me, I'm always the first to question things that seem too good to be true. But, take it from both Rob's experience and my own. A happy, healthy and balanced life is not too far off if you just keep on CUSPing it.

* * *

CHANGES YOU CAN MAKE IN YOUR LIFE TODAY:

- Attempt to follow the MyPlate guidelines for the majority if not all of your meals—just a reminder in case you need it:
  - ½ of your plate filled with fruits and or veggies

- ◆ ¼ of your plate filled with starch
- ◆ ¼ of your plate filled with protein
- Get over your cheese phobia
  - ◆ It's time to stop buying those pre-shredded packs though; shred your own cheese
- Stop pretending you serve yourself healthy portions when you have no regard for the height of your food
- Allow yourself to snack every few hours
  - ◆ But follow the CUSP method to choose a balanced and portioned snack
- Give into those dessert cravings
  - ◆ Always, always, always portion
  - ◆ Ask yourself if the option in front of you is worth it
    - ▪ Will it really satisfy you?
      - ► If yes, go for it!
      - ► If no, hold off until next time
  - ◆ Try buying individually wrapped candies and just having one or two
  - ◆ Remember the first few bites are the best anyway
- Reflect on the way balancing your nutrition makes you feel—peaceful and happy, right?
  - ◆ Apply this balance to all areas of your life :)

PART 6

WHERE WE CAN GO FROM HERE

I hope it's pretty clear to you by now that over the past century in the United States there have been many societal changes that have had devastating effects on our health. But, it would be very unfair to point out flaws without recognition of the many improvements that have also taken place.

Now more than ever people purchase and eat local and organic produce, 100% whole-wheat products, and low sugar alternatives. Fewer and fewer people smoke cigarettes, and more and more people are exercising consistently.

But, we still have a long, long way to go. Even with all these positive changes, obesity rates are still on the rise. Eating whole grains doesn't do much if you eat four servings of pasta at once. Low sugar snacks don't make up for the six cookies you ate after a deprival diet, and exercise simply cannot make up for poor nutrition. We need to make changes today, so that our children, grandchildren, and their future children do not have to live in a world where watching friends and family die of health-related cancers and diseases is anything but uncommon.

CHAPTER 19

THE IMPORTANCE OF HABIT FORMATION

IN THIS CHAPTER YOU WILL LEARN:

- The positive impact healthy eating habits can have on all areas of your life
- The positive impact a consistent exercise routine can have on all areas of your life
- The importance of taking study and work breaks
- How difficult changing habits can be
- The power of Tiny Habits

* * *

Mark looked back over the past few months and could not have felt more proud of himself. He really did it. He transformed his whole life for the better, and it all started with his eating habits. A few months ago, he was sick and tired of feeling sick and tired. His grades had slipped, and he was constantly stressed. He used to eat chicken fingers or pizza at almost every meal and far more dessert than he even enjoyed. By focusing on bettering his eating habits little by little (including more veggies with his meals, not overeating the starch of a meal, only eating dessert until he felt satisfied, etc.) Mark noticed enhancements in many areas of his life.

The first thing he noticed was improvement in his energy level and his sleep schedule. These changes were noticeable after just a few days of a more balanced diet. He could focus better during class and felt like he was absorbing much more information than he had been in the past. For the first time all semester, Mark felt hopeful that he would be able to not just pass his classes, but actually do well. Along with this, he found that he was more alert and productive when studying in the evening. The best part was, when he left the library and headed home, he fell asleep as soon as his head hit the pillow. Mark couldn't even remember the last time that had happened.

Once he noticed this progress, he wanted to do more. So, Mark began including daily exercise in his schedule as well. It seemed so counterintuitive to him. He was taking about an hour per day away from studying, but was somehow doing better in his classes. I hope that I am not the first person to break this news to you, but taking breaks actually increases productivity.

University of Illinois Psychology Professor Alejandro Lleras studied a person's ability to focus and perform a specific task in a one-hour period. He found that unlike those who were required to work straight through the hour and saw performance decline, participants that were allowed to take two brief breaks from the main task produced steady performance throughout the hour.

Exercising during these breaks is even better because it often helps reduce anxiety and stress. Side note- I'm sure most people (myself included) take study breaks and work breaks on our phones, often on social media. This sadly is not a very helpful break, as it can lead to being more tired and can even cause additional stress or anxiety. I know we love our phones, but seriously, go for a walk or something instead. Look at your phone after you're done studying or you've clocked out of work.

Mark started to feel more confident in himself as so many things were going well in his life and on top of that, his body was looking very strong from his challenging workouts complimented by his balanced diet. To his surprise, he started getting more attention from a girl named Michelle he had been interested in since his freshman year. Mark and Michelle started dating and have been together for over two years now.

Mark is extremely lucky. He caught his bad habits early and was able to commit to changing them. I give Mark so much credit because once bad habits form, changing them is a nightmare. In fact, it took me about nine months (that's how long it takes a baby to grow before birth—that's a LONG time) to break my previously unhealthy habits. Whether Mark realized it or not, he was following the CUSP method and applying it to all areas of his life. The CUSP method saved Mark, and it can save you too.

If you have been trying to make a change, and progress isn't going as quickly as you had hoped it would, or if you are deciding right now as you read this that you will start this very second (and I mean this very second, not tomorrow. The whole "I'll start my diet tomorrow" encourages binge eating on the last night of freedom. It's one of the worst things you can do for yourself. But, I know you won't do that. Because you're not going on a diet. You're focusing on a more balanced lifestyle- as corny as that sounds) don't be too hard on yourself. Change takes time. But I promise you, it's worth it.

Follow Mark's example, and start now. Make a conscious effort every single day. Try following the Tiny Habits technique of BJ Fogg, Director of the Persuasive Tech Lab at Stanford University. It's a quite simple framework that has led to behavioral change for thousands of people. It goes something like this, "After I [existing habit], I will [new tiny behavior]." Fogg uses the example of how Tiny Habits can improve your exercise routine. After I go to the bathroom, I will do two pushups. Slowly, you can increase the number of push-ups you'll do. By the end of the day, those pushups will really add up.

Before you know it, your healthy, balanced lifestyle has become second nature. You've probably lost a couple of pounds too, and I would bet all the money in my bank account (well, a lot more than that considering that number is only double digits—I'm a college student remember) that you are your happiest self, just like Mark and so many others who've committed to their health can attest to.

* * *

CHANGES YOU CAN MAKE IN YOUR LIFE TODAY:

- Do you want to be happier, more alert, more productive and experience better sleep?
    - Commit to following the CUSP method for a well-balanced and portioned lifestyle
    - Commit to a daily exercise routine
- Take brief breaks when studying or working—you will get more done in the end
    - Don't take these on your phone—you will get less done in the end
    - Instead, walk around the office or library for some exercise

- Don't give up
  - Habit change takes time, but it's totally worth it
- Never again say you will start your healthy lifestyle tomorrow
  - Or next week
  - Or after lunch
  - Or January 1st
  - Start this very moment
  - The CUSP method is simple, easy and not a diet
    - You don't need to have one last hurrah meal of 5,000 calories
    - Anything you crave fits into CUSP
      - Just keep it balanced and don't overeat
- Try incorporating Tiny Habits into your daily routine
  - Fill in the sentence below with one new habit you want to cultivate
  - "After I [existing habit], I will [new tiny behavior]"
    - Ex: my new tiny habit is—After I brush my teeth, I will do 25 sit-ups
      - That's an extra 50 sit-ups a day I wasn't doing before

CHAPTER 20

THE ALL-YOU-CAN-EAT PLAYBOOK

IN THIS CHAPTER YOU WILL LEARN:

- How poor layouts of dining halls and all-you-can-eat buffets proliferate unhealthy choices
- How making unhealthy options a little less convenient lessens how many people actually go out of their way for them
- How making healthy options a little more convenient increases how many people actually choose these options
- How these same standards of convenience and health can be applied to the layout of your kitchen at home
- Why smaller plates, bowls, serving utensils, and portions need to be implemented into cafeterias

- Why you need to advocate for change in your school, your child's school, or the local school in your community

* * *

Kate entered the dining hall in a bit of a rush. She wanted to get to the library as soon as she could because she had her first midterm of college (and ugh, it was economics) at 8 a.m. (even more ugh) the next morning. The first table she saw as she entered was the dessert table. She grabbed a cookie so she wouldn't have to get up later for one. Kate then glanced at her options.

She really didn't want pasta because she knew it wasn't the best choice before a night of studying. She wanted to memorize her notes at the library, not fall asleep. But, her time was limited and there was only one employee working at the stir-fry vegetable and brown rice station, which was her first choice. On the contrary, there were four employees at the make-your-own pasta line, so that line was moving at about four times the rate of the stir-fry line.

While Kate was waiting in the pasta line, she eyed up the HUGE bowls that students who had just been served were walking away with (talk about overly sized portions). "Why is there no option to choose a smaller bowl size?" Kate thought to herself. It was her turn and she watched in slight disgust as the employee piled on scoop after scoop of spaghetti. It was definitely enough for three separate dinners, but she knew that once it was in front of her, she would end up eating most of it, because it has happened many times before. "Enjoy your meal," the employee smiled and handed Kate the overly sized portion of pasta. Kate faked a smile back. As she walked away, she sighed to herself and thought, "I guess that's just how college dining halls are."

This should absolutely not be the case. Obviously, there is a need for change. This need for change is not limited to only college dining halls; it expands to school cafeterias from pre-k to high school, corporate cafeterias, and other all-you-can-eat buffet restaurants. Kate's same problems occur in all of these places.

Although there have been many efforts in cafeterias in recent years to improve the variety and quantity of healthy options, the nutrition does not make a difference unless people actually eat these foods. And unfortunately, when the choices are a salad bar or a bacon cheeseburger, far too many people go with the bacon burger. And quite frankly, I can't blame them. The burger requires no wait time. It's already cooked and easy to grab as you walk by the station. The salad bar requires me to craft my own salad, and sometimes I just am not in the mood to do that. Convenience goes a long way.

How can these cafeterias create change? It's actually very simple: reduce the subconscious motivators. Make it simple for people to eat healthy. Just like the CUSP method does for you, we need cafeterias to do that same thing for everyone.

Let's look at Kate's first problem: a lack of convenience of healthy options. Why was the first thing that Kate saw when she entered the cafeteria the dessert station? Wouldn't it be easy to move this station to the back or side, making it just a bit more of an effort to grab that cookie?

Dr. Wansink studied how the placement of chocolate milk in one elementary school could lead to an increase in consumption of white milk. He explains, "We never tell them they can't have chocolate milk—that backfires. We just make them think twice about whether they really want it bad enough to wait twenty extra seconds." The chocolate milk was placed in an inconvenient location behind the white milk. With this small change, 30-40% more children drank white milk. This was in comparison to other elementary schools that banned chocolate milk altogether and found that 10% less children drank milk overall and 29% more white milk was taken only to be not touched and thrown away.

Cafeterias should apply this lesson towards many of the unhealthy foods they offer. Don't ban them because #1) it's unrealistic that any food service company will do this.

Unhealthy foods make them money. #2) it won't actually help people eat better. Instead, it will anger them that you took away their freedom of choice. (Plus, we know that not listening to what your bodies are in the mood for leads to overeating in the end anyway—That's where the first letter of CUSP originates).

Make the healthier options the easiest and most convenient to choose and the less healthy options more inconvenient and time consuming to choose. If the dessert table was in the far back corner, Kate wouldn't have grabbed that cookie, but because it was right in front of her—why not?

This is great news for your kitchen at home as well. Purchase all the junk food that you dream about at night. As we know, deprivation doesn't work, and not buying your favorite cookies at the grocery store is very similar to not stocking the cafeteria with chocolate milk. The effects are pretty opposite of good intensions. So buy those goodies, but don't make them readily accessible. Instead of leaving the Tastykakes as the centerpiece of your kitchen table, try a bowl of fruit. If you or someone in your family is really in the mood for those Tastykakes, they'll go to the back of the cabinet where you store them and put in that extra effort. And that's perfectly fine. Let them enjoy it when they are really craving it. But, for the majority of times when they could go for something after dinner, an apple that's right in front of them will probably do the trick.

What would have been the effect if Kate instead saw a table of fruit, not dessert, when she first entered the dining hall? It's pretty likely that she would have chosen a piece of fruit to start off her meal. How can we help Kate continue to make healthier choices out of convenience? The next step is to move the salad bar. By making it impossible for students to get to the other foods without walking around the salad bar, Wansink increased salad sales 200-300% within a few weeks at a school in Lake Placid, New York. He takes the idea of making healthy foods convenient and pushes it a little further. Actually make it inconvenient not to choose the healthy foods.

Kate saw this problem reflected in her cafeteria when there were four employees on the pasta line but only one on the veggie stir fry line. The allotment of employees should be the complete opposite of what it was. Make the healthy options the lines that move the quickest. Kate would have opted for the veggies and brown rice instead of the pasta if that would have been the case.

But, even if Kate chose the veggies and brown rice, she would still have an issue with the obnoxiously large bowls. The portion of rice would have been way too large, and Kate still would have eaten too much (you cannot follow CUSP without portions). In addition to altering the layout and convenience of healthy foods, the other big change cafeterias need to make is in their dinnerware choices. Smaller plates, bowls, and cups absolutely must be incorporated into all cafeterias. Further, the guidelines for MyPlate should be so blatantly obvious that they glare each person in the face with every scoop of food he or she puts on his or her plate. Serving utensils should be smaller throughout the cafeteria, except for at veggie stations or the salad bar where cafeterias should continue using the same size or even go larger.

Another simple change cafeterias can make to size portions down is to serve smaller portions. For example, instead of the slice of pizza that is so large it fills my whole plate, cut that slice in half. Those who only wanted "one slice" will now be consuming only half the calories. This can be applied to the majority of foods and treats in the cafeteria. Mini brownies, smaller chicken nuggets instead of large tenders, and four-inch subs instead of eight. These small changes (literally reducing food portions) will add up, and save the cafeteria a great deal of money too. Oh, and that problem of food waste, you'll see it begin to shrink pretty quickly. It's a win-win-win-win for everyone.

Changes like this make following the CUSP method almost mindless because of how easy it becomes. When the portion is already sized for you, you don't have to think about it. You can just grab it and enjoy.

We can only win if these changes are actually implemented.

Most of them are free or only at the cost of regular maintenance that happens every few years anyway (like purchasing new plates, bowls, and cups). Still, change does not happen overnight. It happens when a group of passionate people join together for a powerful cause.

If you're a student, advocate for these changes to be made in your cafeteria. Let your voice be heard, because you are the one who will directly benefit. Parents, speak to the administrators of your child's pre-k, elementary school, middle school, high school or college to see what improvements can be made in the cafeteria. If your university or school district is managed by a food service company, take the initiative to request continuous improvements (and remember to recognize all the wonderful steps they have already taken in your school or your child's school). Community members, speak up at school board meetings. Take action today so that your loved ones do not have to face the same challenges that Kate did.

∗ ∗ ∗

CHANGES YOU CAN MAKE IN YOUR LIFE TODAY:

- In a dining hall, all-you-can-eat buffet or corporate cafeteria:
  - Don't choose the unhealthy options simply because they are convenient; Instead listen to your body and CUSP it
    - Choose the smallest plates and bowls that are available

- Create your own portions if the ones in the cafeteria are too large
- Always follow the MyPlate guidelines for a balanced meal
  - Take the extra time to wait for the healthy option even if it is less convenient, your body will thank you
- In your kitchen at home:
  - Make healthy foods the convenient ones
    - Keep fruit within eyesight on your table or counter
  - Make unhealthy foods the inconvenient ones
    - Store less healthy foods in a harder to reach and out of sight place, like in the back of a cabinet
  - Always serve pre-portioned amounts of food to make following CUSP as simple as possible for your family
  - Use small plates, bowls, and serving utensils
    - However, with veggies, stick to the same size or even upgrade to a larger size
- Advocate for change in:
  - Your school or university
  - Your child's school or university
  - The school or university nearest to your community

CHAPTER 21

MAKE HEALTHY FOODS COOL (NOT AGAIN BECAUSE THEY NEVER WERE)

———

IN THIS CHAPTER YOU WILL LEARN:

- The positive impact your healthy decisions can have on others
- How positive pressure advertisements can influence social change
- If you do not have your health, you have nothing
- Why we need to encourage those we love to follow the CUSP method

* * *

Anna and her friends sat at their favorite booth at a local eatery on campus. It was a popular spot for students and the girls usually treated themselves about once a week. The place had everything: salads, burgers, tacos, pasta, really anything the girls were ever in the mood for. And, everything was delicious.

Anna wasn't sure what she wanted today. Her roommate, however, was absolutely positive that she was ordering the apples, pears, quinoa and grilled chicken salad. It was her favorite combination. By the time the waitress greeted the table, all of Anna's friends also decided on the salad. "Sure, I'll get the salad too. Why not?" Anna thought to herself.

Remember our friend Samantha? All of her friends ordered burgers and fries so she ended up doing the same. Anna is in the exact opposite position. This is great news. This means that in the same way we can negatively influence the food choices of those around us, we can also positively influence them.

A great example of this phenomenon in the U.S. is in the cigarette industry. Images like the one below, from Complete Wellbeing Publishing, swept the nation following the 1946 Surgeon General's Report on smoking and lung cancer. Efforts like this one helped reduce the number of adults who smoke cigarettes in the U.S from about 42% in 1965 to only 15% today.

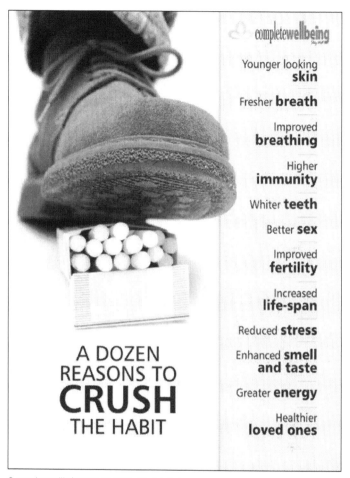

completewellbeing

Younger looking **skin**

Fresher **breath**

Improved **breathing**

Higher **immunity**

Whiter **teeth**

Better **sex**

Improved **fertility**

Increased **life-span**

Reduced **stress**

Enhanced **smell and taste**

Greater **energy**

Healthier **loved ones**

A DOZEN REASONS TO **CRUSH** THE HABIT

© completewellbeing.com. Re-used with permission.

These anti-smoking campaigns exerted a positive pressure to be healthy. We can use this same pressure to help those around us become a little healthier, just like Anna's friends subconsciously did. But, we can make it a conscious effort. It's not just about weight loss, although everyone who is a little self-conscious about having one too many belly rolls would agree that losing a few pounds is a nice added perk. Still, it's about so much more than that. It's about living a long and happy life.

We all want to be there for the "big moments" in life. For college kids like myself, there are many moments ahead of us in both the near and far future: graduation, job, wedding, kids etc. (I could fill this whole page up for just millennials-so I'll spare you). For parents: your child's first steps, first day of school, first time leaving you for college, first time moving into their own home etc. For grandparents: the first time your grandchild says your name, their first sleepover at your house, the day they tell you about their first boyfriend or girlfriend and you wonder where the time went, and eventually the birth of a great-grandchild.

Think of the person you love most in this world. We all have one. No matter what point you are in your life, picture your dream for the future. The grandest goal you've ever thought up. You know that if you achieve this goal, it will be the happiest day of your life. You also know that when you achieve it, that person will be standing right next to you telling you how proud of you they are. Do you have the picture? Good. Now, picture that the person who you love so much is no longer next to you. Does the success taste as sweet? I know mine doesn't. It's an awfully morbid thought and one that I never want to put in my mind again. But it's a necessary thought. Many of us think that we are invincible. That we can drive as fast as we want, drink as much alcohol as we want, eat as much cake as we want, and nothing will ever happen. But it's far from the truth. Every ounce we put in our bodies impacts our health. And our health is something to never take for granted.

The more we follow the CUSP method and eat balanced and well-portioned meals, the lower risk we have of developing deadly cancers and diseases. We know what it feels like to lose someone we love. It is terribly painful to watch them suffer and even more painful inside our hearts. So do not let poor eating habits and a lack of exercise be the reason you and someone you love must suffer in the future.

The power is in our hands to transform the world we live in. We can be like Anna's roommate and encourage those around us to eat healthier through our own enthusiasm. It's time we take responsibility to make health a priority in this country. Instead of trendy deprivation diets becoming viral on the Internet, how about suggestions for balanced meals and exercise tips "break the internet." Or, positive pressure ads like cigarette ones that inform millennials of the many diseases and cancers they may be at a higher risk for simply because of the XXL portions they consume. Let's make the CUSP method the coolest way to eat. Because I think it's really cool to love your body and nourish it, instead of depriving it.

I've created an Instagram account, @cusp_it to use the expansive power of social media to truly make America healthy. Spread the word to friends and family. The time is now to join the CUSP movement.

* * *

CHANGES YOU CAN MAKE IN YOUR LIFE TODAY:

- Order balanced meals when eating out with friends and family
    - And encourage those you love to do the same
- Put positive pressure on the people around you to be healthy
    - They might just need a little push—we all do sometimes
- Remind that one person you love most in the world, that their health is important to you
    - Share with them this book so they can implement the CUSP method for a simple answer towards better health
    - If you can influence them to change just one thing, let it be shrinking those portions
        - In the end, portions can be what nourishes our long lives or sadly cut our lives years too short
            - It's time for you to decide

* * *

Please share this book with that one person you love the most, to help them implement a healthier, happier, and more balanced lifestyle, so they can do everything in their control to be standing right next to you when all your dreams of come true. The power is in your hands to change the world. I cannot do it alone. I need your help. Please, do not let me down. And don't forget to CUSP it.

JOIN THE CUSP MOVEMENT TODAY!

REFERENCES

———

INTRODUCTION: ONE GIRL'S STORY

1. Cusp. merriam-webster.com. https://www.merriam-webster.com/dictionary/cusp. Accessed December 29, 2016.

PART 1: HOW WE GOT HERE

1. Wansink B. *Mindless eating: why we eat more than we think.* New York: Bantam Books; 2006.

CHAPTER 1: THE "FINISH YOUR PLATE" MENTALITY

1. Hunger statistics. wfp.org. https://www.wfp.org/hunger/stats. Published 2016. Accessed November 1, 2016.

2. Wansink B. *Mindless eating: why we eat more than we think.* New York: Bantam Books; 2006.

CHAPTER 2: GROWING PORTIONS + GROWING PLATES = GROWING BELLIES

1. Bhasin, K. Fast Food Burgers Are Now Three Times Larger Than They Were In The 1950s. businessinsider. com. http://www.businessinsider.com/fast-food-burg-ers-are-three-times-larger-than-in-the-1950s-2012-5. Published May 23, 2012. Accessed December 23, 2016.

2. The New (Ab)normal. cdc.gov. https://www.cdc.gov/ nccdphp/dch/multimedia/infographics/newabnormal.htm. Published October 22, 2008. Accessed October 15, 2016.

3. Van Ittersum K, Wansink B. Portion Size Me: Downsizing Our Consumption Norms. *Journal of the American Dietetic Association.* 2007;107(7).

CHAPTER 3: THE IMPOSSIBLE CHALLENGE: ESTIMATING SERVING SIZE

1. Brodwin E, Lee S. Something we have no control over could be playing a huge role in weight gain. businessinsider. com. http://www.businessinsider.com/how-much-have-food-portions-increased-2016-4/#the-staple-city-break-

fast-1. Published April 8, 2016. Accessed October 10, 2016.

2. Optical Illusions. sciencekids.com. http://www.science-kids.co.nz/pictures/illusions/verticalhorizontalillusion.html. Published July 8, 2016. Accessed November 5, 2016.

3. Serving Sizes by Hands. www.wellness4ky.org. http://www.wellness4ky.org/serving-sizes/. Accessed October 1, 2016.

PART 2: CONCENTRATE

1. Wallin P. Why You Want What You Can't Have. selfgrowth.com. http://www.selfgrowth.com/articles/Wallin22.html. Accessed December 15, 2016.

CHAPTER 4: FREEDOM OF CHOICE

1. Wansink B. *Mindless eating: why we eat more than we think.* New York: Bantam Books; 2006.

CHAPTER 6: THE TIME CONSUMPTION CORRELATION

1. Miller, C. How Long Does It Take Your Brain to Register That the Stomach Is Full? livestrong.com. http://www.livestrong.com/

article/480254-how-long-does-it-take-your-brain-to-register-that-the-stomach-is-full/. Published August 16, 2013. Accessed November 15, 2016.

CHAPTER 8: THE DISAPPEARANCE OF SPORTS

1. Probability of Competing Beyond High School. ncaa.org. http://www.ncaa.org/about/resources/research/probability-competing-beyond-high-school. Accessed November 8, 2016.

CHAPTER 10: THE DANGERS OF EMOTIONAL EATING

1. Emotional Eating vs Mindful Eating. helpguide.org. https://www.helpguide.org/articles/diet-weight-loss/emotional-eating.htm. Accessed November 15, 2016.

2. Hartley, R. Emotional Eating is Okay. Really. avocadoadaynutrition.com. http://avocadoadaynutrition.com/2016/11/emotional-eating-is-okay/. Published November 30, 2016. Accessed December 4, 2016.

3. Talens, D. Avoid Emotional Eating with the Broccoli Test. lifehacker.com. http://vitals.lifehacker.com/avoid-emotional-eating-with-the-broccoli-test-1692256729. Published March 19, 2015. Accessed December 1, 2016.

CHAPTER 13: WHAT INSPIRES HEALTHY HABITS?

1. Calculate Your Body Mass Index. nhlbi.nih.gov. https://www.nhlbi.nih.gov/health/educational/lose_wt/BMI/bmicalc.htm. Accessed December 10, 2016.

2. Meet the Millennials: Insights from the 2015 Food and Health Survey. foodinsight.org. http://www.foodinsight.org/2015-food-health-survey-millennial-research. Published October 21, 2015. Accessed September 30, 2016.

3. Overweight and Obesity Statistics. niddk.nih.gov. https://www.niddk.nih.gov/health-information/health-statistics/Pages/overweight-obesity-statistics.aspx. Published October 2012. Accessed November 3, 2016.

4. Ruderman N, Chisholm D, Pi-Sunyer X, Schneider S. *American Diabetes Association.* 1998; 47(5), 699-713. https://doi.org/10.2337/diabetes.47.5.699. Published May 1, 1998. Accessed December 5, 2016.

5. The 2015 Food & Health Survey: Consumer Attitudes toward Food Safety, Nutrition & Health. foodinsight.org. http://www.foodinsight.org/2015-food-health-survey-consumer-research. Published October 21, 2015. Accessed September 30, 2016.

CHAPTER 14: THE DARK SIDE OF SOCIAL MEDIA

1. Meet the Millennials: Insights from the 2015 Food and Health Survey. foodinsight.org. http://www.foodinsight.org/2015-food-health-survey-millennial-research. Published October 21, 2015. Accessed September 30, 2016.

2. Schuble, J. instagram.com https://www.instagram.com/dcfoodporn/?hl=en. Published August 7, 2016. Accessed December 1, 2016.

3. Schuble, J. instagram.com https://www.instagram.com/dcfoodporn/?hl=en. Published July 26, 2016. Accessed December 1, 2016.

4. Schuble, J. instagram.com https://www.instagram.com/dcfoodporn/?hl=en. Published September 22, 2016. Accessed December 1, 2016.

5. Wang GJ, Volkow ND, Telang F, et al. Exposure to appetitive food stimuli markedly activates the human brain. *Neuroimage*. 2004;21(4), 1790-1797.

CHAPTER 15: STRESSED IS DESSERTS SPELLED BACKWARDS

1. Breeze, J. Can Stress Cause Weight Gain?. webmd.com. http://www.webmd.com/diet/features/

stress-weight-gain#1. Accessed September 18, 2016.

2. College cafeteria snack food purchases become less healthy with each passing week of the semester. food-psychology.cornell.edu. http://foodpsychology.cornell.edu/research/college-cafeteria-snack-food-purchases-become-less-healthy-each-passing-week-semester. Accessed November 5, 2016.

3. Glover, L. 6 Reasons for Eating Healthy. nerdwallet.com. https://www.nerdwallet.com/blog/health/medical-costs/benefits-of-eating-healthy/. Published February 12, 2016. Accessed December 15, 2016.

CHAPTER 16: THE DANGEROUS CYCLE

1. Alcohol: If you drink it, keep it moderate. mayoclinic.org. http://www.mayoclinic.org/healthy-lifestyle/nutrition-and-healthy-eating/in-depth/alcohol/art-20044551. Published August 30, 2016. Accessed December 8, 2016.

2. Body Weight Planner. supertracker.usda.gov. https://www.supertracker.usda.gov/bwp/index.html. Accessed December 20, 2016.

CHAPTER 17: BREAKING NEWS: DIETS DON'T WORK

1. Added Sugars. heart.org. http://www.heart.org/HEARTORG/HealthyLiving/HealthyEating/Nutrition/Added-Sugars_UCM_305858_Article.jsp#. Accessed December 17, 2016.

2. Diet Coke Exposed: What Happens One Hour After Drinking Diet Coke, Coke Zero Or Any Other Similar Diet Soda. therenegadepharmacist.com. http://therenegadepharmacist.com/diet-coke-exposed-happens-one-hour-drinking-diet-coke-coke-zero-similar-diet-soda/. Accessed December 15, 2016.

3. Park, A. The Case Against Low-Fat Milk is Stronger than Ever. time.com. http://time.com/4279538/low-fat-milk-vs-whole-milk/. Published April 4, 2016. Accessed December 1, 2016.

4. Starchy Vegetables. md-health.com. http://www.md-health.com/Starchy-Vegetables.html. Accessed December 15, 2016.

5. Wansink B. *Slim by design: mindless eating solutions for everyday life*. New York, NY: HarperCollins Publishers; 2014.

6. Why Do We Need to Eat Fat?. eatbalanced.com. http://www.eatbalanced.com/why-eat-balanced/why-do-we-need-fat/. Accessed December 17, 2016.

CHAPTER 18: USDA'S GENIUS GUIDELINES

1. MyPlate. choosemyplate.gov. https://www.choosemyplate.gov/MyPlate. Accessed September 15, 2016.

2. Why Are Healthy Snacks Important?. healthyeating.sfgate.com. http://healthyeating.sfgate.com/healthy-snacks-important-6727.html.

CHAPTER 19: THE IMPORTANCE OF HABIT FORMATION

1. JD. The Power of Tiny Habits. sourcesofinsight.com. http://sourcesofinsight.com/power-tiny-habits/. Accessed December 31, 2016.

2. Nauert, R. Taking Breaks Found To Improve Attention. psychcentral.com. http://psychcentral.com/news/2011/02/09/taking-breaks-found-to-improve-attention/23329.html. Published February 9, 2011. Accessed December 1, 2016.

CHAPTER 20: THE ALL-YOU-CAN-EAT PLAYBOOK

1. Wansink B. *Slim by design: mindless eating solutions for everyday life.* New York, NY: HarperCollins Publishers; 2014.

CHAPTER 21: MAKE HEALTHY FOODS COOL (NOT AGAIN BECAUSE THEY NEVER WERE)

1. A Dozen Reason's to Crush the Habit. completewellbeing.com. Accessed November 15, 2016.

2. Current Cigarette Smoking Among Adults in the United States. cdc.gov. https://www.cdc.gov/tobacco/data_statistics/fact_sheets/adult_data/cig_smoking/. Accessed December 4, 2016.